C000164510

MAGIC KETO: WHY IT IS CELEBRITIES' FAVORITE DIET?

Embrace The Low-Carb Lifestyle, Eat Exquisite Meals, Burn Fat Like Crazy and Experience Unbelievable Changes in Your Body in Just 30 Days

Table of Contents

Introduction

Congratulations on purchasing this book and thank you for doing so!

The following chapters will discuss what the Ketogenic Diet is and how women can get the best results out of the diet. We will go over what constitutes good fats and bad fats, how to calculate your macros, and how to overcome common mistakes made on this diet. The information found in this audiobook will best explore the adaptations a woman needs to make in order to successfully attain the metabolic state of Ketosis.

Thanks again for choosing this obook! Every effort was made to ensure it is full of as much useful information as possible. Please enjoy!

Chapter 1: What Is the Ketogenic Diet, and How Does It Work?

The Ketogenic diet (Keto, for short) is a diet that heavily reduces the number of carbohydrates (carbs) a body takes in and replaces it with fat. This low-carb, high-fat diet has been studied and has shown to help people lose weight and improve health. There are many different forms of the diet, but the standard Ketogenic diet (SKD) is the most studied and the most widely used. This diet forces the body to burn the intake of fat instead of carbohydrates.

This is how the diet works. If you were to eat a meal rich in carbs, the natural body process would take these carbs and turn them into glucose. Glucose is a sugar that is made to be a primary source of energy to all living things. It is also an integral part of a carbohydrate. Insulin is then produced to move that glucose into the bloodstream to burn for energy or body fuel. Insulin is a hormone produced by the pancreas to regulate and control how much glucose is in the bloodstream. Hence, not having enough insulin causes a form of diabetes.

On the Keto diet, things change. While the process stays the same, the carb intake is very low. Consequently, the body has to utilize another form of energy—and that is where the high-fat part of the diet comes into play. To replace the loss of carbs in the body, the liver takes the fats and turns them into Ketones as its source of energy.

Ketones and Ketosis

Ketones are now byproducts of the body breaking down fat for energy when the carb intake is low. Technically, there are three types of Ketones the body uses on the Keto diet. Acetoacetate is the first Ketone created when the body begins to break down the fat instead of carbohydrates. Acetoacetate is simply created from the process of burning fatty acids. It acts as a taxi or shuttle bus to push the body into Ketosis—much like the beta-hydroxybutyric Ketone. The acetoacetate Ketones form either the beta-hydroxybutyric Ketone or the acetone

Ketone. The beta-hydroxybutyric Ketone (BHB) is not quite a Ketone, but for the sake of the Keto diet, it is considered one. BHB is the most bountiful Ketone in the body, making up over 70% of Ketones in the blood during Ketosis. Here is where we start to see the benefits of the Ketogenic diet—but we will get into those in a bit. While acetone is the simplest Ketone produced from acetoacetate, it is the least abundant. Because BHB is so plentiful, acetone is hardly used as a source of energy. Thus, the body gets rid of it by breaking it down as waste. If a person's body is not using its acetone Ketones to produce energy, you can usually tell by an odor change in the urine or breath. The more a person's breath smells like acetone, the further into Ketosis they are.

Ketosis is a metabolic state formed from raised levels of Ketones in the body. It begins when the body starts to turn its preferred method of using glucose to exert energy to using fatty acids. There are a number of ways to tell if the body is in full Ketosis. The first one is bad breath, which we've already touched on a bit. The acetone Ketones that aren't being used to create fuel for the body are discarded through a person's breath and urine. The most noticeable change is weight loss. The Keto diet rapidly changes the body because the body needs the energy to keep going regardless of what process is being followed. Carbs retain a lot of water—once they nearly disappear from the body, so does a lot of water weight. In consequence, most people in Ketosis see weight changes within the first week. Another way to tell if the body is in Ketosis is having digestive issues. Although these side effects are short-lived while the body adapts to its new course, constipation and diarrhea are pretty common among Keto dieters.

Differences Between the Ketogenic Diet and the Atkins Diet

If you're looking to follow a low-carb diet, both the Ketogenic diet and Atkins diet rank as the most popular. The results are almost identical at first, but the Ketogenic diet began for a completely different reason. It has only recently been used for a weight-loss alternative. The methods behind the diets also differ quite a bit.

The history of the Atkins diet starts off with the founder, Robert C. Atkins. In the 1950s, after receiving his M.D., Atkins started his own practice after a growing concern of prescribed medication as appetite suppressants. The idea of giving medicine to a person to curb their hunger didn't sit well with him. So, he thought of alternative methods. He spent the next decade researching nutrition and carb intake instead of calorie counting, which was a common way of losing weight during the time. He noticed a similarity in reports of the calorie-counting, weight loss method leaving people still feeling hungry. He started a low-carb diet, himself. After noticing a difference, he then had 65 associates go through the same process, all which resulted in weight loss.

The Atkins diet is arranged into four different phases. Phases one is the induction phase—the phase that kicks off the process. The first part of the diet restricts carb intake to less than twenty grams per day while keeping protein and fat input high. Phase two introduces more carbs (between twenty and fifty grams per day). It also suggests more variety of foods, such as more berries, nuts, and vegetables. This is known as the on-going weight loss phase. Phase three is the pre-maintenance stage. It slowly allows a person to add more good carbs to the diet until they become comfortable with the rate at which they are losing weight. And finally, there is the maintenance phase. This is the stage in which the person pursuing the diet reaches their weight loss goal. They only take in the number of carbs that allows them to maintain their weight.

While the Atkins diet results in similar weight loss as the Keto diet, Keto is less structured and easier to follow. Originally, the Keto diet was introduced in the 1910s as a way to control epileptic seizures. It became more popular in the 1920s. The intermitted fasting proved effective as epilepsy therapy. The diet and fasting techniques exhausted certain toxins in the body that researchers believed caused the seizures. The diet became less commonly used with the increased productivity of medications and other sorts of therapy.

The Keto diet revolves around the idea of what the earliest humans would have put into their bodies as food sources. Some would argue that the earliest human's bodies were in a constant state of

Ketosis because of the seasonal food that was readily available to them. There were also states of natural fasting because of the lack of food, altogether. There are no phases in the Ketogenic diet, like the Atkins. Keto allows the individual to start and maintain the weight loss by eating whole foods. Atkins has been criticized by the perception of shakes, bars, and freezer meals that a person needs in order to lose weight.

Keto has also been given credit to more than just weight-loss results. A number of studies result in Keto dieters having enhanced mental clarity and greater levels of energy. Keto is strict with macronutrients and steers a person to balance their macronutrients by eating whole, 'good fat' foods, unlike the Atkins diet. While the weight loss outcomes of the two diets may be similar, to begin with, the Atkins diet slowly reintroduces carbs to the body. This process makes it difficult for the body to maintain the initial weight loss that happens during the induction phase. Keto, however, relies on the same basis of macronutrients throughout the diet. That basis is high calories from fat (70%-80%), moderate calories from protein (20%-25%), and low calories from carbs (5%-10%). This same structure follows the dieter from beginning to end, thus projecting the significance of maintenance throughout the entire process.

The Atkins diet never differentiates on what types of foods can be consumed. It allows the dieter to consume processed foods, as long as it stays within the guidelines of the phase. For example, if you were to walk into a grocery store, you would find sections of aisles dedicated to the Atkins diet. Some of the items include pizzas, shakes, chocolate bars, and even candies. These items are simply low in net carbs (grams of carbs minus grams of fiber). They promote the use of bad ingredients like soy protein and certain sugar alcohols, which have links to other health problems. On the back of any given Atkins bar wrapper, you could also see the use of artificial sweeteners, which have been known to cause more problems than their rivals; natural sweeteners.

The overall goal of Keto is to rid the body of food toxins, which the Atkins diet doesn't address, but rather, promotes in some cases. The Atkins diet allows the consumer to go out and grab a highly processed pack of bacon, and grain-fed, processed meat. Keto emphasizes the consumption of grass-fed, organic meats as well as healthy fats. It strays away from all processed food and relies heavily on foods that are natural but have low levels of sugars, grains, and starches.

Hidden Benefits of the Ketogenic Diet

The benefits of the Ketogenic are vast. We've already discussed some of the benefits, but there are many more! Firstly, the diet increases memory, cognition as well as clarity. Researchers believe that the use of Ketones in place of glucose makes the brain recall events more clearly. Serious studies are being conducted in hopes of deterring early onsets of the Alzheimer's disease. The reason as to why people on the Keto diet have a better mental focus revolves around the idea that carbs as the main energy source give rise and fall to blood sugar levels in the body. This isn't consistent. Hence, it is harder for the brain to stay focused for longer periods of time. When the body switches into Ketosis, using Ketones at its main source of energy, it has a consistent reliance on them to fuel the body at all times. This makes a person focus for a longer period of time. The mind doesn't become clouded.

You also have a more consistent energy pattern. Instead of the energetic ups and downs that come with a high carb intake, your body naturally taps into its unused resources (your fat storage) and provides itself with an even flow of energy. As long as your body is, and stays, in Ketosis, there won't be spikes in your energy levels that are normally caused by increases in blood sugar levels.

The Keto diet is also said to aid in the prevention of some heart-related diseases. Once again, this is due, in part, to the mass reduction and increased stability of glucose levels in the body. Keto dieters have also seen better cholesterol profiles. You might think, a lot of fatty, greasy food is going into your body now, so your cholesterol levels have got to be out of control. A common misconception is that all cholesterol is bad. That is simply not the truth. Cholesterol is a substance made by our livers or comes from the consumption of animal-based products. Whether you consume foods high in cholesterol levels does not necessarily matter because it will always be produced in the liver. The reason the body still produces it is because it is a vital part of the brain and nervous system. Around 25% of a body's cholesterol is found in the brain. It is a building block for some of the connective tissues. Some studies show that people with lower cholesterol levels (below 200) still suffer from heart attacks and strokes. It's actually an overwhelming amount, too. Particularly, a study entitled, The Framingham Heart Study, shows that 40% of its participants that suffered from a heart attack had a cholesterol level below 200. The same study noted that a cholesterol level below 180 actually triples the likelihood of a heart attack or stroke. If a cholesterol level is low, it is a sign of malnutrition. So, a higher cholesterol level is not a bad thing to have, although you do not want it to get too high. You would want to maintain a healthy cholesterol level in your body. The Keto diet, if done correctly, can provide that balance.

Another great benefit of the Ketogenic diet is the decrease of inflammation. Inflammation is defined as the redness, swelling, pain, tenderness and disturbed function to an area of the body. A majority of processed foods break down into glucose. The reduction of glucose metabolism reawakened a protein in the body that suppressed the inflammatory genes. This, in turn, reduced the risks of inflammatory-based illnesses as well as pain.

In addition to these health benefits, the Keto diet also curbs risks of other health-related diseases, like diabetes. Type II diabetes often occurs in adults over the age of 45 who are overweight. With this type of diabetes, the body rejects insulin or simply does not produce enough of it. It may seem strange to suggest a high-fat diet to someone who has type II diabetes, but once Ketosis takes effect and is in sync with the body, it shows great benefits. If you suffer from diabetes, you may want to start the Ketogenic process under the close supervision of a health professional. The switch from using glucose as energy to using fat could be dangerous. Always make sure you test your blood sugar levels while you are on the Keto diet. Sufferers of type II diabetes, once on the diet, notice fewer symptoms. Some even feel the need for less medication. They recognize and adapt to higher insulin sensitivity as well as lower blood pressure levels.

Additionally, the Keto diet improves acne. The modern western diet contains a lot of sugar. Researchers conclude that diet is one of the biggest influences of the prevalence of acne, although it cannot be confirmed. People that eat more whole foods do not have to produce as much insulin as people that eat lots of processed foods. The more insulin the body has to produce, or the more insulin impacts other molecules, the more out of whack the skin becomes. Some of the insulin-impacted molecules create oily sebum. An oily sebum is a fancy term for the wax-like coating that covers pores of hair follicles. It then forms a microcomedone—a clogged skin pore. If the microcomedone is close to the skin, then the skin's pigment will be oxidized by the air, causing it to turn black. If the microcomedone occurs deep within a hair follicle, it will turn white. These are known as whiteheads and blackheads. The formation of these is an ideal place for bacteria to breed, thus inflammation occurs. We see spots of redness, tenderness, and some swelling. The less insulin that is used, the better the skin will be. And to use less insulin in the body means eating whole foods rather than processed foods.

There are many more benefits to the Keto diet. You will feel more alert and less fatigued, and there are a few studies that conclude you will sleep better. Some benefits are still being researched. There are undergoing scientific studies that link better quality of life to cancer patients. Not only that, but some go as far as saying that the diet could greatly impact cancer cells in the body by essentially "starving them" of the glucose they need to grow. While there are no guarantees as of yet, there are some doctors pushing cancer susceptible people, maybe someone that runs a risk of cancer through genetics, toward the Keto-lifestyle.

Chapter 2: Let's Get Started: Ketogenic Diet Food Lists for Women

When it comes to losing weight, it is often harder for women to drop the extra pounds than it is for men. There are particular reasons why, but in general, the female body takes longer to adjust to dietary and lifestyle changes. We will get into the particulars later on. There are specific foods that help kick-start a women's journey on the Keto diet. Women's studies researchers suggest adding more alkaline foods into the diet than recommended. Our bodies have a pH balance that helps us measure the acidity in our blood. If our blood becomes too acidic, it can affect our overall state of health. It is also an optimal place for the growth of illnesses—and even cancers.

The reason researchers push women to eat more alkaline foods is that they contain more nutrients. Foods that are highly acidic have little to no nutrients in them. They promote an array of problems that are meant to be corrected by the Keto diet. Some of those symptoms include:

- Low levels of energy
- Exhaustion
- Acne
- Clouded brain or confusion
- Anxiety
- Joint Pain
- Headaches
- Digestive problems like bloating

The Potential Renal Acid Load scale measures the acidity of a food by a positive, neutral, or negative value. The more negative numbers are the highest alkaline foods. This is not to be confused with the typical, more widely known pH scale. The pH scale is the opposite, which ranges from 0 to 14. The closer to zero, the more acidic a food is. The more alkaline foods are, the closer to 14 they are on the pH scale. Now, let's talk about what types of alkaline foods women could eat on Keto:

Spinach, which has a PRAL (Potential Renal Acid Load: How acidic or alkaline a food is once it's been metabolized) of -11.8. It's highly alkaline and dense in calcium.

Kale has a PRAL of -8.3. Once again, it is highly alkaline and is dense in calcium, iron, and Vitamin K.

Celery has a PRAL of -5.2. Celery is mostly water, which promotes cleansing properties. It can help flush toxins from the body.

Cauliflower has a PRAL of -4.0. Cauliflower is a great food source for Keto-dieting women. It has properties that can aid in balancing hormone levels when they are too high. High hormone levels can have a harmful effect on the body. It can also lead to weight gain, digestive problems like bloating, as well as infertility.

Eggplant has a PRAL of -3.4. Eggplant is also a great food source. It contains phytonutrients like chlorogenic acid. This is a plant compound that helps promote digestion and metabolism.

Zucchini has a PRAL of -2.6. It is a great source of the phytonutrient, lutein, which protects eyesight.

Broccoli has a PRAL of -4.0. It improves skin, metabolism, a healthy immune system and is anti-inflammatory. It also contains a lot of Vitamin K and Vitamin C.

Avocado has a PRAL of -8.2. This is considered the holy grail of Keto dieters. Avocado has a high healthy fat content. It speeds up metabolism and is an anti-inflammatory. It contains a high percentage of Vitamin K, Vitamin C, and potassium.

Bell Peppers have a PRAL of -3.4. They are a powerhouse for decreasing the risks of cardiovascular disease and type II diabetes. They also contain high amounts of Vitamin C, Vitamin A, Vitamin B6, and folate.

Another great food umbrella for women to eat from while on Keto is foods that are high in protein. Protein promotes the release of hormones, which can be a woman's pitfall on Keto, that control appetite. Ghrelin is a peptide hormone found primarily in the stomach. This particular hormone triggers the secretion of growth hormones from the pituitary gland and increases appetite. Eating more protein decreases the amount of ghrelin in the body. Moreover, it actually increases the hormones that help promote a feeling of fullness. A few foods that are high in protein and low in carbs are:

Fish, depending on what type you enjoy, contains a plethora of protein. Some examples of fish to eat that are high in protein and still Keto-friendly are salmon, which can contain upwards of 39 grams of protein per half of a fillet. Let's not forget about tuna. Tuna is a protein powerhouse. It can contain up to 43 grams of protein per half of a fillet.

Chicken is also a good source of protein. Depending on the size of a chicken breast, it can contain around 54 grams of protein per breast.

Eggs are another way to get the daily amount of protein into your diet. A single, large egg has 6 grams of protein.

Nuts also contain high levels of protein. Almonds contain around 20 grams of protein per cup. Pistachios are toward the top of the protein list, containing 25 grams per cup. Hazelnuts are also a great source, containing 20 grams of protein per cup.

Peanut Butter is also a moderate source of protein. Per 2 tbsp. of peanut butter (32 grams), there are 8 grams of protein.
Jerky is an easy way to get a source of protein. It can contain upwards of 9 grams per ounce of jerky (28 grams).

The good thing about foods such as peanut butter and nuts is that they are an easy on-the-go snack. They can easily be eaten by themselves. They can also be paired with other foods. Easy on-the-go, portable snacks can include:

- Peanut butter and celery

- Mixed nuts; trail mix not containing fruits or chocolate pieces
- Hard-boiled eggs
- Jerky sticks
- Cheese Slices
- Dippable veggies

These snacks and many more are great for a woman with a busy lifestyle that still wants to be a Keto dieter!

What Are Good Fats and Bad Fats?

The term good fats sound sort of oxymoronic but there is such a thing! To fully understand what a good fat is, we have to look at all types of fat and what makes them either good for you or bad.

There are three types of fat. Those include saturated, unsaturated, and trans fats. The most notable to avoid is trans fats. There are two types of trans fats found in food. Some of those, but not most, are naturally occurring trans-fat. Naturally occurring trans fats are produced inside an animal's gut and transfer into the foods of said animals. Some of the examples include some red meats and milk. The other type of trans fat is artificial. These types of fats are created by a process in which hydrogen is added to vegetable oils to make them more solid. It is also the most common of the two types of trans fats. The reason it is the most common is simple: it is cheap and easy to use. Trans fats raise the bad cholesterol in your body, which is also known as LDL cholesterol (low-density lipoprotein). This type of cholesterol is what most of us think of as the bad cholesterol in terms of the likelihood of having a heart attack or stroke. It acts as the plaque that clogs arteries.

The easiest way to get trans-fat into your system is by consuming fried and baked foods. Things like donuts, muffins, cookies, cakes, pie crusts, French fries, and biscuits contain trans-fat. The list goes on, but the main culprits can be found in your nearest drive-thru restaurant. You can tell if a product contains trans fats by reading the nutritional label located on most food packages. If a product contains less than .5 grams of trans fat, the producer is not required to label the product as containing it. Sort of scary, right?

Unsaturated fats are also broken down into two categories. The first is monounsaturated fats. This is where you get a lot of your healthy fats. These types of fats can help lower the bad (LDL) cholesterol in your body. Consuming more of the monounsaturated fats also helps lower the risk level of certain types of cardiovascular diseases. While it is not known, some researchers believe that this type of fat can also help control insulin levels and blood sugar. Monounsaturated fats can be found in avocados and avocado oil, olive oil, peanut oil, most nuts, and most seeds.

Polyunsaturated fats are needed in order for the body to function. While they are vital, it is difficult to say whether they are 'good fats' or 'bad fats'. This type of fat can be further divided into Omega-3 fatty acids and Omega-6 fatty acids. Omega-3 fatty acids can be found in fish, flaxseed oil, sunflower seeds, and walnuts. These types of fats are said to be good for the heart.

Omega-6 is debatable. Some believe it is good to help prevent cardiovascular diseases, but not enough is known to determine this as true. Researchers are also unsure of its role as an anti-inflammatory. Omega-6 fatty acids can be found in sunflower oil, soybean oil, and corn oil.

Finally, let's take a look at saturated fats. For years, saturated fats have been seen as harmful. They were said to have increased the risk of heart problems. More recent studies have debunked these myths. In fact, a specific type of saturated fat called medium-chain triglycerides (MCTs) are now known to be digested very easily. Things like coconut oil are MCTs. Once they are eaten, they are immediately passed to the liver and used for energy. They are a great tool to use for weight loss! Saturated fats are known to heighten levels of high-density lipoproteins (HDL). The body needs HDL, or good cholesterol, in order to remove LDL from the body. The more HDL cholesterol you have in your body, the less likely you are to suffer from heart-related diseases. HDL cholesterol acts as a janitor. It cleans the inner walls of your blood vessels, making them healthier. This is important because once the inner walls of your blood vessels become damaged, you are more susceptible to have a heart attack or stroke. While saturated fats increase your levels of HDL, they also take small, dense LDL and make them bigger and less dense, which is good. They do not affect the overall blood lipid profile like the previous thought.

Proteins to Enjoy and to Avoid

If you are looking to start the Ketogenic diet, there are certain foods to enjoy and to avoid. The next few sections will go into depth about what sorts of macronutrient-rich food you should eat. We've already touched on a few examples, but these sections will go deeper into what your diet could look like while on Keto. Variety is important, so let's get started.

Protein is a huge part of the Keto diet. It makes up between 20% and 25% of the foods you should eat. It is essential in the building of muscle and protecting it, regulation of hormones, tissue growth, and the immune system. Here are some proteins to enjoy while on the Keto diet:

- Seafood – most seafood are high in protein and contain very low amounts of carbs, if any.
  – Catfish, cod, flounder, tuna, salmon, trout, mackerel, mahi-mahi
- Some vegetables – some vegetables are low in carbs and high in protein. Steer away from vegetables that contain starches.
  – Cauliflower, broccoli, bell peppers, spinach, some mushrooms, eggplant, celery
- Cheese – there are hundreds of types of cheeses. Virtually all of them are low in carbs and high in protein. They are also good sources of fat!
- Meat and Poultry (grass-fed) – most meat and poultry are considered staples of the Keto diet. There are hardly carbs, if any, and they are also a rich source of protein.
  – beef, chicken, duck, lamb, pork, turkey, ham, deer
- Eggs – eggs are ideal for the Keto diet. They are less than one carb and have around 6 grams of protein.

- Greek Yogurt and Cottage Cheese – both of these items contain a higher number of carbs (around 5 grams) but are healthy and high in protein. They also create the feeling of being full.

Here are some proteins to avoid:
- Whey Protein – whey is a protein that comes from milk. It can also be formed as a byproduct of cheese-making. Whey is highly insulinogenic. Insulinogenic means of, relating to, or stimulating the production of insulin. The entire goal of the Ketogenic diet is to make insulin levels, as well as blood sugar levels, stable and low. Consuming whey disrupts the stability given to your insulin levels while in Ketosis. Some researchers believe consuming whey protein triggers an effect of insulin spikes much like the consumption of white bread.
- Tilapia – Surprisingly, tilapia, while it is a great source of protein, might not be as healthy as you might think. Its ratio of Omega-3 fatty acids to Omega-6 fatty acids concerns health professionals, for one. However, there are thoughts that tilapia also may lead to inflammation.

The Food and Drug Administration (FDA) has also released reports of concerning farming practices when it comes to tilapia. The United States gets most of its tilapia from China, where fish-farming practices include feeding fish other animal feces. This is not to say that tilapia is not a good source of protein, or not healthy because it is. But tilapia need very little nutrition to survive. China provides the United States with over 70% of its consumer-ready tilapia. Another report released by the FDA was said that over 187 shipments of tilapia contained harmful chemicals and pesticide additives. One of these additives is named Methyltestosterone. Methyltestosterone is essentially a steroid that aids the tilapia in its growth. While most countries have banned this additive, the United States still allows it.

- Too much protein – Consuming too much protein can actually kick your body out of Ketosis. If you eat an access to protein, it can actually raise your insulin levels. Your body will recycle the excess protein you do not need and turn it into glucose in a process called gluconeogenesis.

- Cold cuts of meat with added sugar – While some cold cuts of deli meat might be okay on this diet, you have to read labels. A number of deli meats contain additives such as sugar or corn starch. Sugar is what you want to avoid on this diet. Cornstarch is used as a thickening agent to plump up deli meats. It makes them last longer. Cornstarch is used as a replacement of flour in some recipes. Most measurements of cornstarch are cut in half when replacing the flour. So say a recipe contains one cup of flour, you would only use half a cup of cornstarch. Even then, half a cup of cornstarch is over 58 grams of net carbs with little to no dietary fiber to help you knock that number down. It would immediately knock you out of Ketosis. This isn't to say that deli meat is bad on the Keto diet, because they are a great source of protein, but watch the labels and read the nutritional facts before purchasing them.

- Protein is an essential part of this diet, but it is very important to still watch what you are putting into your body. Things such as whey protein, tilapia, and cold cuts of meat are just a few ways bad types of protein can make its way into your body. Also, you don't want to eat too much protein. Be mindful of what sorts of ingredients, rather than foods, you are eating and placing inside your body.

Carbs to Enjoy and to Avoid

A lot of foods we think of as healthy or healthier alternatives actually contain carbs. For example, we think of vegetables as generally healthy. Sure, they have a vast amount of nutrients. But they also contain a lot of carbs. And you want to avoid those as much as possible while doing Keto. It is impossible to avoid all carbs, which is why the Keto diet offers a set amount of carbs per day. The lower intake of carbs, the better off you will be and the faster you will get your body into Ketosis.

Here are some examples of carbs you should enjoy:

- Leafy vegetables – some vegetables are low in carbs. Steer away from vegetables that contain starches. A good rule of thumb is to stick to vegetables that are grown above the ground.
  – Cauliflower, broccoli, bell peppers, spinach, some mushrooms, eggplant, celery
- Nuts and Seeds – they are low in carbs, all-the-while contain high levels of fiber, nutrients, and fats.
  – Almonds, pistachios, hazelnuts, pecans, brazils, macadamia
- Berries – some of the fruits that you can consume while on the Keto diet are berries. They are lower in carbs than other fruits and they also add antioxidants to your diet. Be careful, though, an excessive number of berries can pile on carbs quickly.
  – Strawberries, raspberries, blackberries, blueberries (in moderation), plums
- Fiber Supplements – this is an indigestible carb that guides the digestive system into regulating blood glucose levels and immune system functionality.
  – Acacia, Psyllium Husk
- Avocados – This single food item needs to be categorized by itself. This fruit, while it may be higher in carbs than the previously listed foods, is a Keto staple. It is both high in fiber and high in fat. A single avocado can contain as little as 10 carbs but as much as 17 carbs per avocado. The good thing about this food is the net carbs. Because an avocado is high in fiber as well, it is lower in net carbs, all-the-while still containing upwards of as much as 22 grams of fat! It also contains vitamins such as zinc, iron, and magnesium. It is a great low net carb food.

Now, of course, with the good comes the bad. The 'bad' thing about these types of foods is they are potentially good for you but not on the Keto diet. Here are some bad carbs you'll want to avoid:

- **Grains such as wheat, rye, and corn.** These grains are things we have grown up with; things that we feel when we eat, we are being healthy. When it comes to Keto, this is the group of foods you want to keep away from.

– bread, pasta, cookies, cakes, pizza, buns
- **Legumes such as beans and soy.** They are good for you, in small quantities, for a nutrients supply. Legumes have been around forever, but there is a huge carb intake that comes with eating legumes. Eating a single cup of beans, for example, can have upwards as much as 40 carbs and only 15 grams of fiber. That still leaves you with 25 net carbs. And based on whichever Keto diet you are doing, or however many carbs you are allowed per day, this could be your entire serving!
  – chickpeas, beans, peas, soy
- **Root vegetables such as carrots.** Root vegetables contain way more carbs than vegetables grown above ground. This does not mean these vegetables are 'bad' for you as they contain many nutrients. But they are definitely higher in the carb count. It is safer to avoid these types of vegetables.
  – carrots, onions, parsnip, beetroots
- **Starchy vegetables such as potatoes.** Once again, these vegetables are not 'bad'. They are simply higher in carbs than leafy green vegetables.
  – potatoes, corn, squash, pumpkin, yams, sweet potatoes, plantain
- **Fruits such as apples.** These types of fruits are not only higher in carbs, but they also contain sugar. Sugar can cause spikes in insulin in the body. It is easier just to avoid high sugary fruits.
  – apples, mangos, bananas, watermelon, peaches, oranges

These lists have a lot of foods listed on them, but it is not all of the foods you can eat on the Keto diet. There are plenty of low carb options to choose from. On Keto, variety is important.

Snacks to Enjoy

The Keto diet is one of the most satisfying diets for women. The types of foods that are consumed are relatively filling. Because of the regulations of hormones, blood sugar, insulin and ghrelin it is less likely to become hungry in between meals. That is not to say that it will not happen because it can. It is just less likely. There are a number of high fat, low carb, high protein snack options. Here are some of them:

High-Fat Snacks:
- Avocados – Are you tired of hearing about them, yet?
- Olives
- Pork rinds – These are a good alternative to crackers or chips if you are in that, 'can't just have one' mindset.
- Macadamia nuts
- Dark chocolate – Yes, you can have a Keto-friendly chocolate. It's hard to avoid chocolate, especially when you have cravings. Just make sure this snack has 80% or more cocoa content. The carbs could add up rather quickly.
- Pepperoni slices – Although they are super high in fat, they are highly processed so eat them sparingly.
- High-fat cheeses
- Peanut butter

High-Protein Snacks:
- Sardines
- Beef Jerky
- Cheese chips – a few brands actually make cheese chips. They are crispy chips made out of cheese rather than flour, like a cracker.
- Veggie sticks, like celery
- Hard-boiled eggs

More Low-Carb Snacks:
- Cherry tomatoes – You have to be mindful of how many tomatoes you eat because they do have some carbs.
- Keto chips – They do have added sugars, so you have to be mindful of how many you are eating.
- Guacamole
- Fat Bombs – Fat bombs are quick and easy snacks you can make at home.
- Deli meat and cheese wraps – Once again, be careful when selecting your deli meats.

- Nut butter
- Bone Broth
- Bulletproof coffee
- Sunflower seeds
- Cottage cheese – in moderation
- Pumpkin seeds
- Pickles
- Meatballs
- Avocado fries

There are different variations of some of these foods. For example, you can make
meatballs a number of different ways. The same goes for things like avocado fries, guacamole, and bulletproof coffee. And this is, by all means, not a complete list of all Keto-safe snacks. This is just a starting point in your Keto journey. There are also different types of foods called 'fat-bombs.'

Fat bombs have been popularized in the last few years. These are small round shaped snacks, usually sweet in nature, that have a high concentration of fat. Some of the ingredients include peanut butter, dark chocolate, nuts, and nut butter. And yes, avocados! They help keep you full while waiting on your next meal. If you are afraid you are not going to meet your total fat goal for the day, make a fat-bomb!

Common misconceptions about what things to drink on Keto are vast. One of the biggest pitfalls is drinking diet soda. Regular soda has been criticized among health professionals for years. It is packed with sugar. So, a lot of people believe that switching to diet soda is better. Sure, it has no carbs, no sugar, and tastes pretty similar to regular soda. But researchers believe that diet soda is actually worse for you than regular soda. It is packed with artificial ingredients, including sweeteners. It contains no protein and no fat and is high in sodium. When you consume a diet soda, the body senses a sweet sensation. It expects to receive high blood sugar and insulin, but it never happens. If you consume a lot of diet soda, these constant mixed signals could trigger a metabolic syndrome or type II diabetes.

A great drink alternative to avoid as much soda as possible is Mio. Mio does contain artificial sweeteners and artificial color as well, but all have been approved as safe by the Federal Drug Administration (FDA) as long as it is in small doses. Mio also provides different types of nutritional value. Some types of Mio have vitamins such as B3. B3 is also known as Niacin. Niacin is known to help treat type I diabetes. It is an essential part of our diet. It's also water-soluble so it doesn't get stored in the body. It is a great source of electrolytes as well. Some believe that Gatorade Zero is an option on Keto. The nutritional level of Gatorade is a bit high, though. A normal bottle of Gatorade has about 35 grams of carbs. A G2 version still contains about 12 grams. And the amount of sugar is a bit much. It can contain upwards of twelve grams of sugar. It is important to read the nutritional labels on such drinks to make sure your body isn't ingesting sugar and carbs that you do not want there. It could knock your body out of Ketosis.

Alcohol on Keto is another big restriction. It is best to use pure forms of alcohol to stay within Ketosis. Things such as gin, rum, vodka, tequila, and whiskey all contain zero carbs. But watch what you mix them with. Or you could drink them straight. Red wines and light beers are also okay. But light beers can pile on the carbs rather quickly. They can each contain upwards of 3-4 carbs per serving. Alcohol is also full of empty calories, which can make you hungry. The body treats alcohol as a toxin, too. So, it may slow down the fat burning process. Your body shifts focus from burning fat to pushing the toxins out of your body. Also, you may notice that you get drunker faster. The alcohol hits your system faster and stronger than it did before when your body wasn't in Ketosis. Typically, with a high carb diet, the body had a glycogen cushion built in to slow the metabolizing of alcohol. Without this cushion, the body has no buffer. So, it is best to limit the amount of alcohol you consume while on the Keto diet.

Essential Ketogenic Diet Guidelines for Women

Females typically have more of a body fat percentage than males. Most of that fat storage difference is because of pregnancies and how the woman's body adapts during adolescence. Women usually have between six and eleven percent more body fat than men.

Most of the fat deposits in a sex-related fashion and revolves around the hips, thighs, pelvis, and buttocks of a woman. After adolescence, fat cells do not typically multiply—rather, they grow. Researchers have noted that it is harder for women to lose weight when first starting on a diet, but usually, the weight loss evens out after about six months. It's hard to stay committed to a diet that doesn't give you fast results. Luckily with the Keto diet, you start seeing results within the first week. That makes this diet easier to stick to.

With this diet, there are guidelines for women to follow. Most of these guidelines are customizable. You have to find what works for you. But because our bodies are, more or less, the same when it comes to fattier tissue and deposit areas, here are some of the guidelines that might work for you!

First and foremost, the change will not happen overnight! You have to give yourself time. Drastically changing your eating habits is hard. Some women on Keto have told their stories, and they are too busy to eat low carb, high fat all the time. They can't go to the grocery store; they have to cook dinner for their families. And let's face it, no one wants to cook two different meals—one for you and one for your family. It's hard, but if this diet is for you, don't be hard on yourself to start because it does get easier. The internet has many different guides to help women when first starting a diet. Some sites also give out beginners shopping lists. Use your tools and realize you are not alone if the Keto diet starts off difficult for you. You mustn't get into a failure mindset, though. There is support!

Next, it is important to listen to your body. A hormone imbalance, for women, can really throw a wrench in your Keto plans. Do you crave sugars before your period? What about salt? Do you have severe PMS? Do you have problems focusing? Is your sex drive low? All of these things could be linked to what is called Adrenal Fatigue. While it is not used as a medical diagnosis, it can explain a lot of what you are feeling. Adrenal Fatigue is thought to be caused by chronic stress. Your body is too busy producing flight-or-fight arousal that it cannot produce enough hormones to feel good. Alternative medicine professionals believe this is a real diagnosis, but current blood testing cannot determine a root cause for Adrenal Fatigue. You may not take this at face value, but the symptoms still exist. This hormone imbalance could trigger a number of different things, like more stress! The adrenal gland is responsible for a high production of estrogen, especially in menopausal or pre-menopausal women. It is also responsible for the production of your stress hormones like adrenaline and cortisol. Cortisol is like your body's built-in alarm system. It is your body's main stress hormone. It works hand in hand with your brain to help keep you motivated and control your mood. If your body produces too much cortisol, because you are under a lot of stress or maybe you're not eating enough, it can throw your other hormones out of whack. Whacky hormones can lead to fatigue, weight gain, and irritability. If you ever feel like you could sleep all day, this could be the underlying problem. Your body is tired. During this period of fatigue or any period of fatigue, your body and brain give up. They cannot keep up with the amounts of stress in your world. Stress can, in turn, blow your body out of Ketosis. Higher levels of cortisol actually increase amounts of insulin in the body. The whole goal of the Keto diet is to lower levels of insulin, as well as many other things. If your insulin levels are lower, you actually lower the amounts of cortisol in your body. Your body then becomes less stressed and balances more of your hormones.

Once you develop your plan on Keto, try to stick to it. The key word here is trying! The most important part of this diet is that your body feels good and safe. If you are full at the end of the day, but you didn't eat enough fat or maybe you are low on protein, it is okay. If you are starving, eat—even if it isn't a part of your plan. Not eating can lead to some infertility issues. The more stress placed on your body, the less healed and nourished it is. This, in turn, sends messages to your body telling it is not ready to carry a child. It is thinking fight-or-flight and that there aren't enough calories to have a child. Your body will fight against you to become pregnant, telling you it isn't safe to have a baby. If your body is in starvation mode, it won't produce hormones.

A part of the Keto diet is intermittent fasting. This is where you cycle between periods of eating and not eating. Most Keto dieters fast while they sleep. If you sleep 8 hours every night, you are fasting without even thinking about it. Some people skip breakfast on their days to fast. Maybe they'll eat their first meal around noon. If you go to bed at midnight, you are fasting for 12 hours. The other part of intermittent fasting is the eating window. Once you have fasted, limit your time to eat in a block of time. If you eat your first meal at noon, maybe your next meal is at eight at night. So, you're eating block is between noon and eight while you are fasting. Hunger is not usually a problem while fasting because your body becomes accustomed to your eating patterns. This isn't to say it might not be a bit more difficult to start, but it will get easier. Some women have had success with drinking bullet-proof coffee, or tea while they are in their fasting stage as long as there are no/low amounts of carbs. There are still high amounts of fat in bullet-proof coffee (and some protein) so while fasting, it sends the message to your body that you are okay, and it shouldn't go into starvation mode. It also sends the message to your adrenal glands that you are safe.

Another key thing for women is to not completely cut yourself off from all carbs. The state of Ketosis is reached differently for everyone. It is more difficult for women because our hormones become chaotic with dietary change. To start the Keto diet, you may want to gradually cut back carbs. This could take two to four weeks, sometimes even more time, depending on how your body reacts. So, every once in a while, ask yourself how you feel. Are you still tired? Are you feeling hungry all of the time? If so, gradually add some carbs back into your diet, and then cut them back down again. You don't want your body to stress, because it creates more cortisol. The more cortisol in your body, the more insulin is produced.

Lastly, you have to know the best time to weigh yourself. The absolute best guideline is to keep it consistent. If you weigh yourself once a week, keep it on the same day at the same time, every time. Most Keto dieters weigh in the morning before eating. If your weight fluctuates a bit, it is hard not to get discouraged. But fear not! If your body is still in Ketosis, it is still fat-burning. The weight differences are usually from the large amounts of water that are needed in this diet.

These guidelines are meant to help. Being a woman on the Keto diet is difficult. There are many things women have to take into consideration that do not mean as much to men. Please remember, these guidelines differ from person to person. And there are many more!

Common Mistakes on the Keto Diet and How to Overcome Them

There are quite a few common mistakes made on the Keto diet. It's hard! You are not only changing your diet; you are changing your lifestyle. It takes a lot of focus and a lot of drive to become fully Ketogenic. Your body is making a change, so you have to follow suit.

Here are some common mistakes that are made on the Keto diet and how you overcome them.

The first is not paying attention to how you feel. There is already some information listed above about this subject, but it's a big enough mistake and needs to be hit hard. A lot of people get caught up in whether or not they are losing weight. What matters is that you are being healthy. This isn't as simple as it may sound. But the truth with this diet is that if you are following guidelines, and you feel good about what you are putting into your body, the initial weight loss will follow.

Secondly, thinking it is all about the food you are putting into your body is a mistake. This sort of diet is a lifestyle change. Of course, you can make healthier eating choices, and you should. Along with the diet portion comes typical weight loss protocols. Exercising is very important. It helps boost along your weight loss journey. Physical activities also reduce the further risks of type II diabetes, cancers, and cardiovascular disease. Increasing the number of physical activities, you do per day also improves your quality of life. So, if you are a victim of the first mistake of not paying attention to how you are feeling, there is a remedy that could potentially help. Exercise can also help you sleep better, lower blood pressure levels, lower levels of bad cholesterol and build stronger muscles and bones.

Thirdly, do not try to force things to happen. Some things work for some people. Not everything that is in this audiobook will work for you. If intermittent fasting isn't up your alley, you do not have to do it. The goal here is to make you feel comfortable with doing Keto, all-the-while eating better and making healthier choices. If something isn't for you, it doesn't mean you can't be on the Keto diet. Sculpt this diet to fit your needs.

The biggest and the most important mistake is being afraid to make mistakes and comparing yourself to others. No two single people are the same or are built the same way. This is especially hard for women. There seems to be a standard that all women have to meet in order to be considered beautiful. While things are changing in the entertainment industry, it is still hard to not compare yourself to someone who is thinner, leaner, or more muscular. You have to do what is best for you. The only comparison to be made is to your previous self. Are you making improvements? Do you feel better about yourself? Are you happier? Are you healthier?

While it is important to consult with medical professionals and listen to what they have to say, it gets hard to determine what to do on this diet. You'll come to find out that doctors, Keto-bloggers, or research students do not agree on most things. If one doctor says to eat more greenery, and another says to eat more meat, what do you do? Try both! See what works best for you and stick to it! You have to do what is best for you and your body. You don't have to pick a side or stance. You can do whatever fits within your life. You can even switch it up after a while and change your mind. Keep all doors and options open with this diet.

Another mistake that is made on Keto, quite frequently, is snacking. Some people think that because there are no calorie restrictions, that they can eat as much as they want. This isn't necessarily true. Snacking can get out of hand rather quickly. Once you are on the diet, find a meal plan that works for you. Find foods that will keep you full longer. A high number of people on Keto don't feel like they need snacks because of how fulfilling their meals are. This may not be true for everyone. But this does not mean you should sit on the couch and eat pork rinds all day. Those calories add up, and simply put—it isn't good for you. A way to avoid this is to plan out a snack. Once you've gotten used to how your body feels on Keto, determine the best time to eat a snack during your day (a time you know you'll be hungry) and eat it. This suppresses the urge to go to your fridge every hour and eat a cheese stick or eat a spoonful of peanut butter.

Another common mistake is constantly striving for perfection. You are going to wear yourself down by trying to hit your macros every day. It is okay to be out of tune every once in a while, as long as you plan to correct it the next day. Being perfect is not sustainable. You might find yourself fasting only three or four days a week, or maybe only hitting your macros three days out of the week and that is okay. If you constantly stress about hitting your goals each and every day, chances are you will burn yourself out. Not to mention, stress could knock your body out of Ketosis. Just do what you feel you can do. If you can only change smaller things to start with, that is good! It is better than what you were doing. And if you feel like it, gradually add more changes to your lifestyle.

Another major mistake people make is falling into a uniformity of foods you can eat. Being on the Keto diet still allows for varieties of foods. You'll want to expand that variety to gain as much and as many nutrients as you can. The cool thing about Keto is if you think of a food that you really want, chances are, there is a Keto version of it. The internet is endless with recipes for Keto dishes and is a great resource to find something new and inventive to eat.

It is very common to not hold yourself accountable. That goes with any diet. Accountability goes a lot further than accepting responsibility for your actions. It is being able to justify why you did something. The thing about not working out for a couple of weeks or eating a cookie every once in a while is that it turns into a habit. While you are on this diet, ask yourself if it is worth it? You have to be honest with yourself. It might be a bit easier if you have been on this diet for a while because the food isn't used for entertainment anymore. It becomes something you need rather than want. If it helps, connect with other people who can support you on your journey. Do have those people who help you hold you accountable. You could join a group on a social media platform. You could do diet bets. Maybe you and a friend, or you and your spouse start this journey together. See who can out-diet who.

Another mistake is not measuring your macros at all. In order to be successful on this diet, you have to know what you are putting into your body. There are numerous apps that you can download to keep track of your macros. Once you have been accustomed to certain foods and how much you can eat, maybe measuring macros isn't right for you. But in order to begin, it is important to know what sorts of foods help you hit your goals.

The last mistake to mention is one that is all too common and is probably the hardest to correct. You simply aren't eating enough fat. Most people have a fat-phobia, meaning they feel like putting too much fat into your body can clog arteries and cause heart attacks. This isn't true. This myth has been dispelled since the 50s. This high-fat diet is just that: high in fat. You have to consume enough fat to make up for the loss of carbs. If this doesn't happen, you could plateau. The same goes with not having enough protein in your diet. This means that after the initial drop in weight, you could go months without losing any more. There is a chance that your macros aren't where they need to be. You have to eat fat! And lots of it!

There are a number of trial and tribulations you need to overcome while on the Keto diet. Listen to what your body is telling you and work with it, not against it. These common mistakes could be costing you a lot more than what you think. But, where this is a will, there is a way. Don't get discouraged if you have been doing some of these things. It's okay. Move forward!

Chapter 3: Tips to Adapt to the Ketogenic Lifestyle

Common Pitfalls Women Face on the Ketogenic Diet and How to Overcome Them

The Ketogenic diet is different for women than it is for men. One of the main reasons is something we have already discussed—hormones. Women are more sensitive when it comes to hormones. We have a cycle that our bodies go through, and being on the Keto diet acts as a healer. Once again, you can't just drop everything that you are eating today and start off with no/low carbs tomorrow. It is a process, and a woman's body is delicate. It takes time to switch a diet and have your body follow up with you to know how you are doing—and the results all depend on how you feel. If you feel healthier, more awake, less fatigued, and less clouded, you are doing something right for yourself.

Some women, once transitioning to the Keto diet, don't get enough electrolytes. That is because there is not as much sodium and potassium in whole foods as there is in processed foods. So once you make the switch, make sure that you find a way to get electrolytes into your system. Not having enough electrolytes in your system can result in a few different problems. One would be cravings. Your body is so used to the amount of sodium, that it craves it once it's not getting any. Cravings are hard to deal with because it can be a "reason to live" so to speak. This means that it controls you, and it is literally all you can think about. Make sure you load up on foods that are high in potassium and sodium. Avocados and spinach are great sources!

When women think about the Keto diet, they begin thinking about the amount of fat they have to eat. When you are basing a high-fat diet solely on fat, you probably aren't getting enough of the nutrient-dense, leafy greens. This is hard because a lot of people know veggies are high in carbs, so they tend to think they should just avoid them altogether. This is not the case. Things such as kale, broccoli, and spinach are essential to this diet to get adequate nutrition into your body.

When you get on the Keto diet, exercise is very important alongside the foods you will be eating. Exercising actually drains your glycogen storage. This is where glucose is stored in the body. Thus, the more you exercise, the easier it is and the faster you get into Ketosis. Always find a way to do a bit of exercise in your daily routine. It could be as simple as taking a short walk with your dog. Try to exercise for around thirty minutes per day.

Another pitfall of women on the Keto diet is forcing the body to fast. In short, if you are hungry, eat. If you are full, stop eating. While the percentages of macros in your diet are important, you have to listen to your body. Don't fast for the sake of fasting. You have to do what is genuinely best for you.

A lot of these problems and mistakes can actually make women last longer in what is called the Keto-flu. There will be more discussion on that later on. It is just important to balance your new lifestyle. Rather than just eating the right types of foods, you have to exercise, replenish key electrolytes, and make sure you are doing only what you need to do—not what everyone else *thinks* you should do.

Does the Ketogenic Diet Suit You?

The short answer to this question is yes. In some form, the Keto diet is a great way to eat and be healthy. Let's go a little more in depth. There are four types of Ketogenic diets, so there are a lot more options for you if the standard Ketogenic diet (SKD) does not work for you.

The second type is called the cyclical Ketogenic diet (CKD). This sort of diet involves two days of heavy carb eating and then five days of the standard Keto diet. If you are super athletic or work out a lot, this may be the type of Keto diet for you. The two days of high carb loading helps refill muscles in order to retain them during rigorous work out periods.

The third type of Keto diet is called the targeted Ketogenic diet. This diet allows you to add carbs just around work out times. It's like a mixture of the SKD and CKD. This allows you to still get the carbs you need in order to retain muscle during workouts, but you are not out of Ketosis for days at a time. It is just short periods of time during the day. If you do moderate workouts and aren't involved in any strength training, then the SKD is what you need.

The last type of Keto diet is called the high-protein Ketogenic diet. This is similar to SKD but overall, it has more proteins and less fat. The ratio often looks like this: 60% fats, 35% proteins, and 5% carbs. This is ideal for people who are looking to build muscle mass or slow the breakdown of it. Most people who are on this diet are bodybuilders and older people. It is also good for people who show signs of protein deficiency. If you have a protein deficiency, it can show by the loss of muscle mass or by thinning hair.

Pick which diet is best for you. Professionals warn about the process of Keto-cycling, though while on the CKD. Keto-cycling is the process of eating carbs and then restricting yourself again. It can be dangerous to the body in terms of fluctuations of body water. These changes can lead to dizziness and can potentially worsen heart conditions. Always consult with your doctor before beginning a diet and determine which one is right for you.

If you are busy and are having problems trying to figure out if the Ketogenic diet best suits you and your life, the chances are it couldn't hurt. If you are looking to increase your overall wellbeing, it is suited for you. If you are looking to lose weight, it is suited for you. If you would like to introduce more nutrients into your diet, it is suited for you. The good thing about the Keto diet is that it could be integrated into any lifestyle. If you feel as if you are too busy to adapt to these changes, no worries. There is no rush. You can slowly integrate this diet into your life. It is actually recommended that you gradually change your eating habits over a two to four-week period.

If you are afraid of being a woman of convenience, there's nothing to fear. It is ten times easier to go through a drive-thru or order a pizza for dinner rather than cooking. But a lot of fast-food places offer Keto-friendly foods. You just have to research what you can eat from these places of ease. The Keto diet adapts to many different types of lifestyles. Find one that works for you.

The Lack of Fiber

Some people fear that with the decrease in carbs on the Keto diet, it will be difficult to get enough fiber into their body. You have to cut out the majority of fruits and all starchy vegetables, so how do you get fiber into your diet? The term dietary fiber refers to the indigestible part of the plant food that travels through our digestive system. Fiber helps prevent constipation as well as protects against heart disease, gastrointestinal health, maintains healthy insulin levels for diabetics, and aids in weight loss.

There are two types of fiber. The first one is soluble fiber. This type of fiber binds together with fatty acids in the body. It is very important to make sure you are eating the right types of foods for this fiber to be prominent in the body. It has a very important function. After it binds to the fatty acids, it slows them down which, in turn, takes them longer to empty out of the stomach. Therefore, you feel fuller for longer periods of time. Furthermore, it also slows down the rate at which the body absorbs sugar. Soluble fiber lowers bad LDL and regulates sugar intake as a whole. This is helpful for people that are diabetic. Some foods that will help you increase your soluble fiber levels are flaxseeds, chia seeds, coconut, spinach, and avocado.

The second type of fiber is insoluble fiber. It helps move solid waste through the digestive tract. It also helps control pH levels in the intestines. This type of fiber has a number of benefits, also. Insoluble fibers speed up the waste removal process of the body. It also promotes regular bowel movements and prevents constipation. Some foods that will help you increase your insoluble fiber levels are cauliflower, raspberries, and broccoli.

Soluble fiber dissolves in water whereas insoluble does not. Insoluble fiber actually never changes its shape as it travels through the digestive system. Soluble fiber does change but never completely breaks down. As it absorbs water, it becomes more gelatinous. Insoluble is stronger and does not break down as it pushes through your digestive tract. Some people think of it as a scouring pad moving through your body. It pushes things where they need to go and cleans up any mess left behind. Soluble fiber makes it harder for your body to break down carbs and process them into glucose. In turn, this lowers the intensity of blood sugar spikes in your body which then, regulates insulin levels.

If your intake of fiber is low, it is hard to satisfy that feeling of being full. Ultimately, because you are snacking more often to feel satisfied, you can potentially reverse your weight loss progress on Keto. It can even knock your body out of Ketosis.

If you have a good amount of fiber in your diet, you can usually tell by not feeling constipated. This differs from person to person. The same amount of dietary fiber is not going to be the same for everyone. So, find a level of fiber that works best with your body. Another important rule of thumb is to drink plenty of water while on Keto. There is a more likely chance that you could become dehydrated as the fiber in your body is absorbing and holding on to water.

Fiber is very important while on the Keto diet. But there are things to watch out for. One of those things is called isomaltooligosaccharides (IMO). IMOs can be made in a few different ways. They are all mostly derived from a sugar called maltose. IMOs are promoted as a dietary fiber with a hint of sweetness. They are predominantly found in nutrition bars, healthy cookies, and candies. The problem with them is that they are promoted as fibers, but do not break down the same way. Once they start breaking down, IMOs can actually turn into glucose and maltose. Because they have to potential to create high blood glucose levels, they could also create spikes in insulin which is what Keto dieters are trying to avoid.

So, what do you need to know about fiber and carbs? When you look at food labeling and notice the term net carbs, it means the total number of carbs minus grams of fiber. For example, if you are consuming a protein bar and it says it has 4 net carbs, but you turn it over and it reads 25 carbs, that means there are 21 grams of fiber in that item. That gives you your total net carbs. Net carbs are tricky though. Before you begin the Keto diet, ask yourself about your goals and what you want to get out of being on this diet. If you are more sensitive to the carb take away that occurs on the diet, maybe measuring net carbs is better for you. Some people who, rather than lose weight, want to maintain it measure their carb intake by using net carbs. Others who may want to lose more measure total carbs. It is up to you, your body and what you can handle. It may even switch for you while on the diet. Instead of measuring total carbs, you switch to measuring net carbs and vice versa.

A lot of dieters forget about fiber, which is why they run into digestive problems like constipation. People get caught up in the low carb, high-fat part of the diet too easily. Always remember your fiber because it can also aid in weight loss. Fiber is a tool that can change and affect bacteria in your gut. The change in bacteria can change the ability to burn fat. There was a specific study done in Canada to confirm this. Doctors took a group of kids who were obese. Half of the kids received extra fiber in their diet for sixteen weeks; the other group did not receive the added fiber. What doctors learned is that the group of children's, who received the extra fiber, body composition completely changed. Their gut microbiomes also changed. Those children lost 2.4% more body fat than the children that did not receive fiber. The take away here is simply not to forget about fiber and your leafy green vegetables. Yes, you need to increase fat intake. Yes, you need to lower your carb intake, but it is important not to do so at the expense of your fiber consumption. Fiber is your friend.

Too Much Protein

Consuming too much protein can be damaging to your body. If you are using protein as a way to lose weight, it can actually make you gain weight in the long haul. That is why it is so important to count your macros. A set amount of protein is essential to almost all diets. It helps repair and strengthen the muscle. It even creates new muscle. It also helps build strong bones, organs, and maintains healthy brain function.

Protein is essential on the Ketogenic diet. There is a process the body goes through while in Ketosis. First and foremost, the body will always, always go for glucose to burn for energy if it is in the body. That is why you minimize the number of carbs eaten in a day. If the body can't get to the glucose that it needs, it will go for muscle protein and break it down in a process called *gluconeogenesis,* which means making new sugar. This is why it is so important to eat enough protein. If you eat a certain amount of protein a day, the body will defer from using muscle protein and resort to using the protein you've eaten in your foods to create new sugar. This entire process is being aided by the fat you are consuming. When the fat burns, the liver releases Ketones and provides the energy to conduct this activity in your body.

How do you know the correct amount of protein to eat in a day? There is a good equation to go by, and that some medical professionals actually recommend. For every pound that you weigh, you would need between .3 grams and .7 grams of protein. So, for example, say you weigh 200 pounds. You would take 200 and multiply it by .3 or whatever amount of protein you think you need. That equals 60 grams of protein per day. You would need more protein (.7 grams) if you worked out regularly.

A regular, consistent source of protein is recommended on the Keto diet. Configure how much protein you need in a single day and find good sources through Keto-approved foods. There is a wide variety of foods and resources to pick from, just be careful not to overdo it. Too much protein can affect your kidneys and cause kidney stones. It can also strain your liver. Make sure you are careful when counting grams of protein. When you are consuming .7 grams per pound of weight, it can become excessive, especially when you are not working out on a regular basis. Excessive protein will also create more fat in your body. The proteins that are not needed to carry out certain functions of the body are converted to sugar.

Protein affects the body differently for women, as well. Women's bodies are on a monthly cycle. Depending on which point you are at on your cycle, proteins can affect Ketone levels differently. During the luteal phase, for example, women are more likely to consume protein and have it not affect their Ketone levels. During a follicular phase, however, that exact amount of protein may decrease

Ketone production. One of the easiest ways to find a personal protein limit is to purchase a Blood-Ketone meter. These are commonly used by people with diabetes and Keto-dieters. The meter does read differently for people on Keto. A normal Ketogenic state will have a reading between 0.5 and 3 mmol/L. It may take some time to get these results but stick with it! At certain points, it may read differently, and that is okay. It all depends on where you are at in your monthly cycle. Eventually, you will get an understanding of when your Ketone levels are good and when they drop a bit—if they do at all. Retaining an adequate amount of protein in your diet and in your body can help you to stay regular.

Dehydration

Your body is over 50% water. When starting a low carb diet, your body experiences loss of water. This is more likely to happen at the beginning of the diet when your body goes through a rapid change it is not used it. So, always be mindful of how much water you need in your diet.

If you feel dehydrated when first starting on Keto, here is why! Whenever you consume a carb, it is stored in the form of glycogen. Glycogen is a polysaccharide (a carbohydrate that has molecules of sugar bonded together) that forms glucose. From there the body automatically stores three to four grams of water. It does so because of glucose spikes levels of insulin in the body. When there is a spike of insulin in the body, the kidneys tell the rest of the body to hold onto water. When you are on a low carb diet, that process does not occur. The kidneys stop sending the signal to the rest of the body. They don't need to hold on to as much water as they did before. So, they tell the body it is okay to get rid of the excess water. This is why people feel better within days of starting the Keto diet. Because you are getting rid of the excess water in your body, inflammation also goes down. There's a reduction in edema. Edema is the medical term for swelling. This is usually caused by sodium. Sodium creates the ability to hold on to that water. On the diet, you are not consuming as much sodium as you used to, so it is easy to see results within days. You may even see a couple of pounds missing from the scale.

Because the kidneys are no longer sending the signal to the rest of the body to retain water, you may find yourself peeing more often. This is a good sign that you are headed in the right direction but it can also go too far. When you urinate, you are not only losing water, you are also losing sodium. Sodium, in this case, is not your average table salt. Sodium is very important for proper bodily function as it contains a lot of minerals. The problem people run into is not being able to replenish the lost sodium. Low carb foods don't have a lot of good sodium in them. So, what happens is that you lose all of the good sodium minerals and replace them with bad sodium minerals. Once this happens, dieters begin losing other minerals like potassium and magnesium. Then you are left with a bad mineral balance. With that, we lose the ability to function on all cylinders. Our nerves do not fire in the proper way. This causes you to feel weak. Your electrolytes are depleted. When you feel weak, your appetite is not there. When your appetite is not there it is harder to drink water.

So how do you overcome dehydration and replenish your body? The first thing is to add some sodium back into your body. This can be done by using Himalayan pink salt or Hawaiian black sand sea salt, or basically any type of sea salt—just not iodized table salt. The first step into rehydrating your body is to increase your sodium. At this point in time, your intake needs to be a little bit higher than normal. Most researchers suggest 3-5 grams of sodium to start off. This will help correct the sudden mineral imbalance your body just went through. If you plan on working out one day, make sure you increase the amounts of sodium before you do so. Once you start sweating, you are depleting your sodium stores. Remember, your kidneys aren't working like they used to. If you don't replenish before you begin your workout, you will resort back to being weaker once you're done, so always eat more sodium before a workout and not after. Plus, the increase in sodium before gives you the energy boost you may need to make it through.

Also, to stay hydrated there is a key thing that you could do. It is drink water. Water is super important while you are on a low carb diet, for the reasons listed above. Dehydration can cause many symptoms that can throw your body out of whack. Some of them are:

- Less frequent urination
- Dizziness
- Confusion
- Fatigue
- Extreme thirst
- Dark-colored urine
- Bad breath
- Constipation
- Dry skin
- Headaches

If you experience any of these symptoms, you may be dehydrated. If you can't get to a source of water and you start to feel any of these symptoms, caffeine is a good source, regardless of what some researchers might say. Caffeine makes you have to urinate, meaning it gives the signs that you may become dehydrated quickly. This isn't the case. There are properties of caffeinated beverages that offset the loss of fluid in the body. This isn't the only way to become hydrated quickly, though. Here some ideas on how to hydrate quickly.

- Eat something salty
- Eat raspberries or blueberries
- Lie down (conserve energy)
- Eat broth
- Eat Greek yogurt
- Drink fresh coconut water
- Green smoothies
- Eat water-rich vegetables

Make sure to listen to your body and watch for signs of dehydration, especially while your body is going into Ketosis. It's hard to determine if your body is dehydrated, but hopefully, these tips help out. This is not a complete list of what dehydration looks like or feels like, but it could give you a sign while you are on the Keto diet.

What is the Ketogenic Flu, and How to Get Over It?

If you are starting to research the Ketogenic diet, you might come across terms such as 'Keto sickness,' or 'Keto virus.' These are all referring to the most common use of its name, the Keto flu. There are many symptoms associated with the Keto flu. They much resemble influenza. But there are reasons why your body is acting like it is sick. And truthfully, it is but you are working toward a healing process.

The first reason your body is acting like it's sick is that you are going through a withdraw. Eating carbs, sugars, and things alike triggers the reward system in the brain. Having those things in your system releases dopamine. Dopamine is a neurotransmitter responsible for sending messages from your nerve cells to your brain. When your body doesn't receive the sugar and carbs that it is used to, those messages are not sent. Your body has a negative response. Sometimes, it goes as far as being depressed and getting irritable.

Another part of the Keto flu is best explained using an example. When you are burning through the last of the carbs in your body, you feel okay. But you haven't tapped into the best source yet. Think of your gas tank on your car. You have regular old fuel in there and its only goal is to get you from point A to point B, but you also have a reserve can in your trunk, which is filled with premium fuel. However, you can't use it until all of your regular, unleaded fuel is gone. Much like an empty gas tank, there is sludge that can build up on the bottom. This happens when you don't clean your tank out regularly and water and trash start to build up—much like your body when you begin Keto. You are cleaning out the last of the bad 'sludge.' When you are going through the Keto flu, your body is using up the last of its sludge. It's nearly at the point of running out of gas, but not quite yet. It still has enough to run, but barely. Once you run out of the sludge, then you can start using your premium gas. In this case, it is going to be your stored fat. That is the good stuff, and that is when your body jumps out of its depressive, fatigued state. It begins running off of fat instead of carbs and glucose.

Another part of the Keto flu is a mineral deficiency. Because your body is used to having the carbs and glucose run the show, it has a specific process that it goes through to create energy. On the Keto diet, that process has to change. Your body is learning something new and needs time to adapt, much like any other diet. But one thing your body is not doing is regulating sodium and water. It will learn the new steps eventually, but during the Keto flu portion of the diet, it isn't keeping up. Your body is losing a lot of sodium and water all at once. And it's hard to replenish them. Your body is becoming dehydrated. Because your minerals are so low, you are also experiencing an electrolyte deficiency. If you feel nauseous while experiencing the Keto flu, this would be why. The three most important electrolytes to focus on are sodium, of course, magnesium and potassium. There are ways to quickly replenish those electrolytes!

To quickly elevate levels of sodium:
- Bouillon cubes—drop your favorite flavor into a hot cup of water and dissolve it. Each of these could contain upwards of about 2100mg of sodium which is almost half of what you need to make it through the day
- Salt shooter—you could place Himalayan pink salt or a brand of sea salt in a glass of water and mix it with lemon or lime juice.

To quickly elevate levels of Magnesium:
- It is easiest to use a supplement that provides you with your daily need of magnesium.
- Eat avocados!
- Snack on some nuts
- Snack on some seeds

To quickly elevate levels of potassium:
- Eat avocados!
- Eat spinach
- Eat mushrooms

To fully regain all of these electrolytes remember to use an optimal cook method where you are not wasting any of the vital nutrients. If you are cooking mushrooms or spinach, a lot of the nutrients could come out of the broth. So make sure you are eating, and maybe sipping, as much as you can!

Another big part of the Keto flu is caused by the switch from carbs to fats in the gut. When we switch it up, our body begins creating endotoxins because there is too much fat being used at once. Endotoxins are toxins that are present inside of a bacterial cell. It is released when a cell disintegrates which allows them to thrive whereas our gut bacteria has to take a back seat. Endotoxins are also sometimes responsible for mimicking symptoms related to certain diseases. When these endotoxins are released into the bloodstream, the gut bacteria become out of whack and doesn't know what to do in the beginning. The bacteria in our gut is so used to carbs, so once you start throwing fats at it, it has to have time to adapt. The types of bacteria that feed on fat are good, but they have to get ready to thrive.

An easy way to get through this transitional phase of the Keto flu is to drink bone broth. Bone broth is incredibly powerful when it comes to healing the gut. It contains collagen which reduces inflammation and helps heal the intestinal lining. Plus, it's easy for the gut to digest and retain all of its minerals and proteins.

Another part of the Keto flu is your body producing too many Ketones. It is still in its transitional phase and is learning how to adapt to what you are putting into it. The best way to get rid of the excess Ketones is to burn them off. Light cardio is a great way to help your body get through the Keto flu. While transitioning into the Ketogenic state, you and your body have to work together. It makes the Keto flu easier to deal with.

Types of Supplements to Help You on the Ketogenic Diet

There are a number of supplements on the market to help you along on your Keto journey. Supplements are not necessary, but they are helpful when you may not get enough of an electrolyte in your system, or enough of a mineral in your system. They do come in handy. Here are some supplements that might help you.

- Magnesium, potassium, and sodium supplements—these could help you when you are going through the Keto flu. Furthermore, they might become a staple that you take all of the time when you are living your Keto life. It depends on you and how you feel. If your body is low on electrolytes or maybe you know you didn't eat what you needed to eat in a day, these supplements might be a good idea for you.
- Different types of sea salts—if taking a sodium supplement isn't for you, you can experiment with different types of sea salts.
- Fish oil—it puts omega-3 fatty acids into your body that you would normally get from fish. If you are not a fish person, this may work for you. It helps balance those omega-3s and helps to put fat nutrients into the body. Fish oil can aid in weight loss, and for women, it can help with period pains, breast pains, and even pregnancy pains. It's a good general supplement that can make your Keto transition easier.
- MCT oils—these are helpful for the body and to make its job less strenuous. MCT oils are made from coconut oil or palm oil. Coconut is preferred for Keto dieters. But it is an immediate source of Ketones because it glides through the gut into the liver and is either converted into energy or it is converted into Ketones. It also promotes healing to the body.
- Vitamin D—while this one isn't necessary, it is a good idea to have this on hand. Most Americans are Vitamin D deficient. Having a sufficient supply of Vitamin D in your body supports facilitating the absorption of calcium, which is a nutrient that could be lacking in the Ketogenic diet.
- Exogenous Ketones—if there comes a point where you fall off of the Keto diet, this supplement could help you get back into Ketosis faster by providing an outside source of Ketones to your body.

- Keto Green Blend—this could be a number of different things. It is a pill or powder that supplies all (or most) nutritional value that you would otherwise get from leafy green vegetables.

These supplements are just ways to help you succeed on Keto. They aren't necessary, but they are helpful. And some of the help you break out of the Keto flu faster. So, if that is something you are not looking forward to, something like a multivitamin with sodium, magnesium, and potassium could help your transition.

Types of Supplements to Help You Get Over the Ketogenic Flu

These supplements are going to be sort of the same as the Ketogenic Diet Supplements. The same types of supplements that will help you get over Keto flu will aid you on the Ketogenic diet. These include magnesium, potassium, and sodium supplements. MCT oils will help you out as well. You always want to make sure that you are replenishing your body with enough electrolytes and water as your body transitions from carb-burning to fat-burning. You also want to make sure you are drinking a lot of water. The electrolyte supplements are really going to help you overcome the Keto flu. When you begin to feel sick or nauseous it is because you have an electrolyte imbalance. You are quickly losing a lot of your stored nutrients, so you have to make up for it by either taking supplements or eating foods heavy in potassium, magnesium, or sodium. MCT oils are also a great way to begin healing the body. While the body is starting to use Ketones, you can take an MCT oil. It will quickly hit your liver and produce energy or convert to Ketones.

The best 'supplement' you can use is exercise. A light cardio workout is a great tool to help you get over the Keto flu. It doesn't have to be strenuous, but any physical activity will aid you.

Avoid Nutrient-Poor Fat Bombs

Let's refresh on what exactly a fat bomb is and what it is going to do for your body. A fat bomb is essentially a tool to help curb your appetite as you wait for your next meal. They are becoming more popular with the Ketogenic lifestyle as people refrain from eating between meals. These simple, small, circular shaped balls of fat are a great way to avoid over-eating in between meals. Rather than prioritizing protein or other essential nutrients, they prioritize fat, helping you stay full for longer periods of time.

The dangers of fat bombs come into play when you have no self-control. Also, a lot of fat bombs have stuff like nuts in them, which contain a lot of protein. Remember, if you overeat protein it could knock you out of Ketosis. So, putting so much fat and sweetness into a candy-like state could be dangerous. You also want to make sure you are putting the right ingredients into your fat bombs. With these types of 'snacking' foods, you will want to make sure you are really loading up on the fat. These bombs are not supposed to be high in protein. If they are high in protein and fat, it'll take your body even longer to burn the fat that is already inside of your belly or on your butt or thighs. The idea of a fat bomb and why it is so small is because your body can quickly burn off the new fat that just entered, and then continue to burn the rest of the fat that is already there. It is sort of like a jump start. While this is happening, though, you aren't hungry and are hardly thinking about food. This deters you away from snack searching, too. Just grab a fat bomb!

How to Make a Fat Bomb as Nutrient-Dense as Possible?

If you are wanting to make a fat bomb and gain some nutrients while you eat it, there are certain ways to make them. They are a bit more strenuous when it comes to making them, but they are beneficial. These fat bombs can actually be a meal replacement.

First, these fat bombs are more intricate and have more ingredients than the common three or four it takes to make a regular fat bomb.

All fat bombs, though, have a base. Most bases are something that is super high in fat like coconut oil, cream cheese, or butter. On top of the base, you have to add your nutrient-dense ingredients. Herbs and spices are a good way to get some nutrients into your fat bombs. Some spices, like cinnamon, are great antibacterial and immune system healers that could prevent and even treat some infections. Herbs, like rosemary, can boost cognitive function just by the smell. Herbs contain a number of minerals, vitamins, and antioxidants.

Some people even add low carb fruits into their fat bombs. Things such as blueberries, raspberries, and lemon juice are beneficial that protect us from heart diseases, and even cancers.

Nuts and seeds are a great source of protein, fat, and fiber that can be added to your fat bombs. Crushing up nuts or using a nut butter to coat your fat bomb is a great addition because all of the sources of nuts make up a greater body composition and improve health.

Fat bombs don't always have to be sweet in nature. There are great recipes for nutrient-dense fat bombs that taste like pizza, salmon, or jalapeño poppers that act as a meal. These are designed to keep you fuller for a longer period of time.

There is also a thing called bulletproof coffee (BPC). This is a lot like a fat bomb and does the same thing. Grab your favorite coffee. It could be literally any type of coffee you enjoy that does not have carbs or protein. Brew your coffee like you normally would and drop a couple of pads of butter in it. Once it melts, stir it in and drink your coffee as normal. This is a great source of fat in the morning if you are working on your intermittent fasting. It helps fill you up so you curb the need to eat. The same thing can be done with teas, also. It immediately gives you energy! If you do not have butter, MTC oil is a great alternative. It is also preferred by some people because it doesn't have a taste. If neither one of these options are easy for you to get your hands on, coconut oil works and so does heavy cream. Be careful with heavy cream, though. It does contain protein so if you are looking to just stick with fat, heavy cream may not work for you. That protein could be turned into glucose and defeat the purpose of drinking fatty coffee or tea. The body will immediately burn the protein instead of the fat.

The good thing about the Keto diet is that you can find or make any variation of food you normally enjoy, in a low carb fashion. Things like fat bombs are designed to satisfy some of those needs for a pizza, or a cookie.

Chapter 4: How to Find Your Suitable Meal Portion

The easiest way to find a meal portion that is suitable to you and your lifestyle is to first determine your macros. If you find that your macros are too high and that you can't seem to fit it all in a day, then try taking supplements in place of some of the macros you are not reaching. For example, if you are not meeting your protein goal, maybe try a protein powder in a nutrient-dense shake.

There are a number of ways to make sure your meal portions are adequate for the Keto diet. If you find that you can't meet your fat intake, there are simple ways to add the fat into things you normally drink or eat. For example, the BPC is a great way to make sure that the fat gets into your diet. Coffee is something you would normally drink, right? Adding the grass-fed butter or MCT oil will increase your fat intake.

Meal portions are essential in making sure that you enter your correct macros for the day. There are a number of apps that can help with this. MyFitnessPal is a great way to track macros, and it is pretty simple to use. The KetoDiet app is another great way to track your macros. This app also lists recipes by the thousands! So if you are afraid you are not getting enough variety in your diet, this application could be great for you! There are more apps you could download and use. Some of them are listed below.

- Carb Manager
- Total Keto Diet
- Senza
- Cron-O-Meter
- FatSecret
- Wholesome
- Ketosense
- Zero

These apps hold different things as a priority. You should download an app depending on what you think is most important to you. These will help you determine your meal portions. Once you get on a diet, it is hard to figure out what you can and cannot eat. These apps will help you determine your daily intakes. Once you figure that out, you can determine how much you should be eating during what meal. If you have a light breakfast, or no breakfast at all (intermittent fasting), you will be able to eat a heavier dinner or lunch. These meals should meet your daily macros. If you eat a heavy lunch, maybe your dinner is lighter. A majority of your carbs should be eaten in the morning as well, especially before a workout. That way, you are burning them off throughout the day. As a side note, if you eat heavier fats during breakfast or lunch, or maybe a heavy snack, you will find that you are not as hungry at night. Therefore, you'll eat less. Your body will burn stored fat while you sleep rather than the fat you just put into your body.

One of the biggest mistakes made on Keto is thinking that you can just eat lots of meats and cheeses and be okay. That is not the case. A good purchase to keep in mind when starting this diet is measuring cups. To accurately determine macros, you'll need accurate portion sizes. A food scale also works in this circumstance. It will guide you in determining what meal portions are suitable to meet your macros.

Practice Good Eating Habits

It is important to practice good eating habits while on the Ketogenic diet. There are dietitians that stress a couple of key points that will get you further on Keto. But once again, listen to your body. If these habits are not working for you, try something else. The thing about this diet is whatever your body says you need to do, is what you should be doing. This can even mean adding back in a few more carbs per day. Or maybe it is eating more fats. It could even be not eating breakfast in the mornings. Just make sure you are listening to your body's signals. Some of the recommended practices are listed below.

- Eat more fiber — a lot of people do not get enough fiber in their diet.

- Eat greener, above-the-ground vegetables.
- Don't deprive yourself of foods you love. This is very important because a lot of researchers believe if you don't eat what you want when you want it, it will come back to haunt you. So, if you want that chocolate bar, eat it. The good thing about Keto is that you can make a Keto-friendly chocolate bar. You can make almost anything you would normally eat, but it won't mess up your diet.
- Consume a variety of foods — this is also very important. If you find yourself eating the same thing over and over, you will probably become bored. If you become bored, it can really mess with your brain. You want to research a variety of recipes. Almost any food can be made in a Keto-friendly manner. Make sure you shake it up a little, try new foods, and stick to your macros. Plus, if you aren't eating a variety of foods, you may not be getting all of the nutrients you need.
- Control your portions — this can easily happen by eating more fats. You will fill up faster.
- Drink plenty of water — sometimes thirst can be misinterpreted as hunger. Try drinking an 8-ounce glass of water if you start to feel hungry and you know it is not time to eat.
- Pay attention to ingredients and know what you are eating — chances are you've eaten a food in the last couple of days and you have no idea what is in it. If a word ends in -ol, it could be a sugar alcohol. Some Keto dieters do not pay attention to sugar alcohol but some of them have the potential to kick your body out of Ketosis. Not only that, but they can make you crave the real thing!

It is important to know what you are putting into your body. If you aren't familiar with an ingredient, maybe you shouldn't be eating it. Do your research and practice eating habits that work for you and your lifestyle. Also, make sure you are drinking plenty of water. Find different ways to make sure you are eating the right amount of nutrients without overeating or increasing your carbs. It is well worth the time it takes to find what works for you.

Calculate Your Diet Macros

The top macros you will concern yourself with while on the Ketogenic diet are fats, proteins, and carbs. When you first start the Keto diet, it is important to calculate your macros. You have to determine what you are putting into your body, and what your shortcomings are. Once you get used to it, however, it might not be for you. A number of apps will help you figure out what works best for you. They will have you enter your current weight and the weight loss goals you are wanting to achieve. From there, you will be given your daily macro goals. You can enter the foods and drinks you consume in a day and it will let you know what you need to work on. For most people, it is hard to initially consume all of the fats you need to on the Keto diet. Calculating your macros will help! Once you have a good idea of where you stand, or maybe you have reached a weight that you are happy with, you want to maintain it. Then, calculating your macros might not be necessary. Until then, this audiobook will recommend that you do.

Your daily macros may different from someone else on Keto and that is okay. You have to determine what works best for you. Everyone's body composition is different. And depending on the goals you want to achieve, macros will differ for everyone. The general rule is that you need to consume 60% fat, 35% protein, and 5% carbs. This could differ depending on your goals. For example, if you are leaner and you want to retain or grow muscle mass, you would eat less fat than those on a standard Ketogenic diet. Maybe your fat goal for the day is 50%. You would eat a lot more protein, also, because you need to retain your current muscle mass and build on top of it. If you are on the Keto diet to lose more weight, then you would consume more fat than someone who is leaner. It all depends on which Keto diet you are on, and what results you are looking for. Listen the section **"Does the Ketogenic Diet Suit You?"** to fully understand which type of Ketogenic diet you are looking for.

Essential Guide on: Ketogenic Diet for Premenopausal Women

There are a number of problems women face as they become premenopausal. Some of those things are hot flashes, mood swings, insomnia, and weight gain. It is the butt end of comedic relief on some sitcoms but being premenopausal is no laughing matter for women who are going through it. This is the transitional period between when a woman goes from having a regular menstrual cycle to not having one. While this change is happening, hormones are erratic. Once a woman hits menopause, insulin levels and blood glucose imbalances can increase the number of symptoms a woman has. Women are busy trying to find alternative therapies when dealing with these symptoms. Following a standard Ketogenic diet can actually alleviate some of the hard to deal with symptoms.

In a woman's body, hormones act as messengers to the rest of the body to maintain chemical and physical functions of the body. As a women ages, her body produces fewer eggs, progesterone, and estrogen. Changes in these hormones can lead to whacky levels of insulin, ghrelin, and leptin. Having lower levels of estrogen can promote spikes of blood glucose levels as well as insulin resistance. Insulin resistance is a process in which the body's cells resist the effects of insulin. The cells begin to refuse glucose, thus spiking levels of blood sugar. This creates a higher production of insulin. Higher amounts of insulin can potentially result in weight gain.

Because women have been conditioned to refuse fat and stick with a high amount of carbs for numbers of years, it is hard to get on the Keto diet. But the Keto diet can actually help women going through the stages of menopause. It can benefit in many ways. Some of those ways are listed below.

- Can control weight gain
- Reduces the risk of cognitive decline
- Stabilizes blood sugar levels
- Improves mood
- Lowers inflammation
- Increases energy levels
- Improve sleep quality

There are other benefits that come with being on the Keto diet, but these are just a few of the most significant changes that can help a woman's transition to menopause.

Essential Guide on the Ketogenic Diet for Women Who Have Type II Diabetes

Diabetes is a problem with your body as it produces higher levels of glucose than normal. Type II diabetes is the most common form of diabetes. If you have type II, your body does not produce insulin normally. At first, your pancreas produces more to make up for the deficiency, but eventually, the body cannot keep up.

If you have type II diabetes, it is recommended that you begin this diet in the hospital. It is extremely important to monitor your blood glucose and Ketone levels when your body makes the transition and begins burning off the last of its carb fuel. Even once your body adjusts to the diet, it is important to regularly check your glucose levels. Follow up visits to your doctor are also recommended. This is just in case your body is not adapting well to the diet or in case you need to make some adjustments.

There have been a number of studies conducted to see the effects of the Keto diet on people with type II diabetes. Participants of the studies have shown greater control of the glucose in their blood and a need for less medication while on a low carb intake.

Still, this diet may not be what's best for you, if you suffer from type II diabetes. People find that this diet is hard to stay on for long periods of time. Yo-yo dieting (going on and off a diet or switching up diets) can be dangerous for diabetics. If you plan on taking a break from Keto, or maybe trying a different plant-based diet, make sure you talk to your doctor before doing so.

There are a number of benefits that type II diabetics have experienced while using the Keto methods. Participants in other studies saw a reduction in body weight, hemoglobin A1C, and glucose levels in the blood. The low carb diet also shows much more

56

substantial results than a low-calorie diet. While a low-calorie diet has shown improvements, the low carb diet has even greater improvements.

Low-Calorie Diet for People with Type II Diabetes:
- 16% blood glucose reduction
- 2.7% reduction in body mass index
- 6.9 kg reduction of body weight (15.2 pounds)

Low-Carb Diet for People with Type II Diabetes:
- 19.9% blood glucose reduction
- 3.9% reduction in body mass index
- 11.1 kg reduction of body weight (24.4 pounds)

People who had undergone the low carb diet versus the low-calorie diet also found a significant reduction in A1C hemoglobin levels. The reduction of hemoglobin A1C in low carb dieters was over 3 times that of the low-calorie diet (0.5% vs. 1.5%). Hemoglobin A1c is the measure of glucose bound to your red blood cells. If your A1C count is high, you have more glucose in your blood. So, the less, the better. The normal range for a person without diabetes is around 4 and 5.6%. If you have a hemoglobin A1C level between 5.7% and 6.4%, you are at higher risk of becoming diabetic. If your level is above 6.5%, you are considered diabetic. When you test for hemoglobin A1C, and you are diabetic, you want your levels to read less than 7%. The higher your level is, the more you suffer the symptoms typical of being type II diabetic. Type II diabetics that used Keto saw a significant drop in A1C levels. The blood cells live for about three months, so a hemoglobin test every three months showed tests results like this: test one: 7.7%; test 2: 6.4%; test 3: 6.4%; test 4: 6.4%.

Essential Guide on the Ketogenic Diet for Women Who Are Overweight

It is a lot harder for women to lose weight than it is for men, especially when first starting a diet. Women may not see results as fast. This is because of the fact that a woman's body stores more fat than a man's. This is a preemptive design given to women because our bodies are made to birth a child. Fat around the hips and buttocks are produced by estrogen. Stomach fat is usually built because of stress put on the body. Flabby arms could be caused by low testosterone levels. The list goes on, but what does the Ketogenic diet do for these specific types of weight gain?

The process of Ketosis can target specific areas of the body. Ketosis affects a woman's hormones different than a man's. It is a lot harder for a woman to stay in Ketosis because they don't immediately see as much in terms of results. But that doesn't mean it isn't working. Ketosis can help regulate a woman's hormones. There is a lot of hearsay about how a Ketogenic diet can ruin a woman's hormones. This simply isn't true. One of the main concerns is the thyroid. Carbs are necessary for thyroid function. If you lower your carb intake, there is a lot less T3 being circulated throughout the body. The Ketogenic diet does promote a less circulated T3 hormone, but a decreased T3 hormone does not mean your thyroid is dysfunctional or that you are suffering from hyperthyroidism. Hyperthyroidism is categorized by a thyroid not producing enough T4 hormones. It has nothing to do with T3. Thus, the change in the amount of T3 being produced by the thyroid does not cause a dysfunctional thyroid. There is another underlying problem if that is the case. Levels of T3 decrease independently on the Keto diet. A lower level of T3 is actually shown to be beneficial to women. It can preserve muscle longer and improve longevity.

Some women say that Ketosis didn't work for them to lose weight. The answer is simple, though. Those women weren't in Ketosis. So, if you find yourself not losing weight like you want to, or your energy levels are not there, double check your macros. See what you are putting into your body. There is a chance you weren't in Ketosis, to begin with.

Another problem, and one that has already been discussed, is that you might not be eating enough. It is hard for women to eat tons of fat because we have been conditioned to not eat it. So there is a high chance that you simply aren't getting enough into your diet to lose weight.

Another problem that women run into is that they are overtraining. If you work out a lot, a standard Keto diet may not be working for you. Try to find a suitable Keto diet that works with your levels of physical activities. You may need to increase the numbers of carbs you eat per day or increase your protein intake. Overtraining while on Keto can really mess with your hormones. It could also mess with your reproductive organs and increase your levels of cortisol. The problem here is that you are using the wrong tool for the wrong job. So, find something that works for you.

In order to effectively lose unwanted weight, you have to make sure you are in Ketosis, or go-figure, it doesn't work. Women's hormones make it a bit trickier to actually know if the diet is working or not. Find out before giving up and always, always listen to your body.

Chapter 5: How to Get the Best Out of the Ketogenic Diet

Combine the Ketogenic Lifestyle with Exercise to Speed Up Fat Burning.

Trying a new work out when first starting Keto may not be such a good idea. At first, your body is still trying to get used to its new process—hence, you won't feel as great when you are finished. That is not to say that working out is not a part of the Ketogenic diet—it can be. It is important to work out while on Keto (although it is not necessary), but take it easy to start with and don't overwork your body. If you are highly active, don't worry—you can still do Keto.

If you are big into cardio, that is a great way to increase the amount of fat you are burning while on Keto. While you are running or biking, since you are already burning fat, it will oxidize. You will use less oxygen and produce less lactate. This could lead to more fat burning during workouts.

The important thing to remember is that your body needs carbs to boost through a workout, so if you are highly active, try a different Ketogenic diet that allows for a higher carb intake. A common myth that is misunderstood is that you have to work out in order to lose weight on Keto. That is simply not true. The standard Ketogenic diet does not involve working out as a part of the weight loss process—but it can truly help. It can also get you over a plateau. If you hop on a scale every Monday to see how much weight you have lost and see that the number isn't getting any smaller, you may have plateaued. If that is the case, add a simple cardio routine into your day. This could help boost fat burning. Revisiting your macros might help, too.

If you are highly active, don't let the Keto myths scare you away from trying it. It is still a great way to boost energy levels, elevate cognitive brain function, and regulate hormones. Keto also won't make your performance suffer. You might think that because you are eating fewer carbs that you won't have the energy to make it through your run. This is false. It might happen during the start of the Keto diet when your body is making the transition between glucose and fat, but it won't stay that way. Athletes who have been on the Keto diet have had the same performance results as they did before.

The best types of workouts for women on the Keto diet are:

- Cardio (Aerobic exercise): a physical exercise that goes from low to high intensity, lasting over a period of three minutes. An example of this is jogging.

- Anaerobic exercise: a physical exercise that consists of short bursts of energy. For a standard Keto diet, this is not a recommended work out. Fat, alone, cannot fuel this type of activity. An example of this is weight-training.
- Flexibility exercise: This is categorized by the stretching of muscles, joints, and getting a better range of motion in your muscles. An example of this is yoga.

- Stability exercise: This is balance and core training. This helps improve your alignment as well as strengthen muscles. An example of this would be doing squats and liftoffs.

Combine the Ketogenic Lifestyle with Intermittent Fasting.

Intermittent fasting is a big part of Keto. It is an eating style where you only eat in a given time frame and then fast the rest of the time. Most people on Keto fast for 16 hours a day and eat throughout eight hours. For example, you eat only from noon to eight at night. After eight, you do not eat anything and fast while you sleep. Then, you eat again at noon the next day. This is the easiest way to fast. Your body also changes quite a bit during this time. Human Growth Hormones (HGH) increase drastically. When these hormones are deficient in our bodies, it can lead to weight gain and decreased bone mass. So, an increase in HGH is beneficial while on the Keto diet. Insulin sensitivity also improves while fasting. Insulin levels drop dramatically which makes stored body fat easily accessible. Our cells can also go through cellular repair during this time. When cells fast, they start cellular repair processes on other cells that are dysfunctional. They can also digest old proteins that build up inside cells. Fasting can also increase the release of fat burning hormones! Fasting has a host of other benefits. But sometimes fasting isn't for you and that is okay.

If you google fasting for women, you might get a lot of people posting backlash to this method. Everyone is entitled to their own opinions but fasting is not bad like some people think. Women may have to fast differently from men as a result. So, don't accept everything at face value and do your own research to determine whether fasting is right for you. Let's take a look at some of the hormones affected by fasting.

- Starvation hormones: women are much more sensitive to these hormones. It is a protective mechanism in place for bearing a child. If your body realizes it is not receiving adequate foods, it won't want to produce eggs. But this is completely natural. This is why some women drink BPC while fasting. It sends messages to the body to tell it that it is okay and that you are not starving.

- Thyroid hormones: this goes back to the myths about levels of T3 and T4. When you are fasting, the thyroid is less active, but it is also less active during periods of time between meals. It is just the natural response. If you are worried about something being wrong with your thyroid, an easy way to tell is if you become cold all of the time.

If you find that fasting does not work for you, come back to it later and try again. It might not work because your body isn't used to it yet. When you fast, certain processes in the body no longer happen because they don't need to. Sometimes it doesn't work right off the bat. So, revisit it later. It might be easier.

Intermittent fasting revolves around the idea of how our ancestors may not have had food sources readily available to them. The process of hunting and gathering only worked if there were sources of food to hunt and gather. Sometimes, they wouldn't eat for a long period of time. That is when they burnt off their stored fat. Stored fat is a great tool our bodies have used since the beginning. If they didn't have stored fat, we might not be here today! But sometimes, that fat makes us look in a way we don't want to be. We used this ability to survive during periods of famine. Fat was the most sensible way to live during these times. Now that we don't live in periods of famine, the fat just builds until we burn it off.

Chapter 6: Recipes, Advice, and Examples

Quick Breakfast Recipes

If you find yourself busy—maybe you have kids and are trying to get them ready for school in the mornings—these are some easy recipes that will satisfy you (Keto-friendly) and satisfy your family. These are just beginner recipes. Thousands of more recipes can be found online.

Avocado Bacon and Eggs (3g net carbs)

Ingredients:
- **One medium avocado**
- **2 eggs**
- **Bacon bits, or cooked bacon**
- **Salt**
- **Cheddar cheese, shredded**

Instructions:
First, preheat your oven to 425 degrees. Begin by cutting the avocado in half and by removing the pit. You'll want to remove some of the insides of the avocado to make the pit hole bigger. However, don't let the avocado go to waste—eat it! Place your avocado half in a muffin pan to stabilize it while you add the egg to the hole. Sprinkle cheddar cheese on top of the egg, along with salt preference. Cover the top of the avocado with bacon bits. Cook in a muffin pan at 425 degrees for 14–16 minutes. Serve warm. If you do not like bacon, sausage can substitute.

Cheesy Sausage Puffs *(1g carb per puff)*

Ingredients:
- 1-pound Jimmy Dean Sausage of any variety
- 2 cups of shredded cheddar cheese
- 4 eggs
- 4.5 tbsp. of butter, melted and cooled
- 2 tbsp. of sour cream
- 1/3 cup of coconut flour (heaping)
- ¼ tsp of baking powder
- ¼ tsp of salt
- ¼ tsp of garlic (optional)

Instructions:
Melt butter in the microwave for 10-15 seconds, then place in refrigerator to cool for 10 minutes. Meanwhile, preheat the oven to 375 degrees, and line a large baking sheet with foil, or some sort of non-stick paper. Begin browning the sausage. Once done, drain it and cut it into small pieces. Set aside. In a medium or large size bowl, begin mixing eggs, butter, sour cream, salt, and garlic. Slowly add the coconut flour and baking powder and stir until it is combined. Mix in the browned sausage and cheese. Roll your batter into one-inch balls and place on baking sheet. They only need to be about a half an inch apart from one another. Bake for 14–18 minutes or until lightly browned. Enjoy! Store the leftovers in the freezer for another Keto-friendly breakfast later in the week. Do not keep leftovers longer than 7 days. If you are craving a bread-like consistency, add another half a cup of coconut flour to make them a bit more bread-like.

Keto Blackberry Cheesecake Smoothie (6.7g net carbs)

Ingredients:
- ½ a cup of blackberries, fresh or frozen
- ¼ cup of full-fat cream cheese, or creamed coconut milk
- ¼ cup of heavy whipping cream or coconut milk
- ½ cup of water
- 1 tbsp. of MCT oil or extra virgin coconut oil
- ½ tsp of sugar-free vanilla extract or ¼ tsp of pure vanilla powder
- Optional: 1-3 drops of liquid stevia or another artificial, Keto-approved sweetener

Instructions:
Combine all ingredients into a blender with the exception of the blackberries. Add the stevia if you would like to. Slowly blend all ingredients together. Once blended, add in blackberries slowly. Continue adding blackberries until ½ a cup is reached. Blend to preferred consistency. Pour in a glass and enjoy!

Quick Recipes for Lunch

Cheesy Cauliflower and Bacon Soup (4.4g net carbs)

Ingredients:
- 1/4 cup of olive oil
- 1 tsp minced garlic
- 1 medium head of cauliflower, chopped
- 2 cups of chicken broth
- 1 cup of water
- 1 cup of heavy whipping cream
- 1 tsp xanthan gum
- 1.5 cups of shredded cheddar cheese
- 4 tbsp. bacon bits

Instructions:
In a deep stove-top pan, heat up ¾ of the olive oil and minced garlic. Once it is hot, add in the medium head of cauliflower, chopped. Keep on high heat. Pour in chicken broth and water and wait for a boil. Stir frequently. Once it is boiling, add in the heavy whipping cream and continue to stir. Bring the heat down to medium. In another bowl, mix the excess olive oil and xanthan gum together until blended. Drop your mixture into the rest of the soup and continue to stir. It should start thickening. Slowly add in your cheese so it has a chance to melt. Pour your bacon bits in, serve, and enjoy!

Chili Lime Lettuce Wraps (1.9g net carbs per leaf)

Ingredients:

Marinade:
- 2 tbsp. of olive oil
- 1 tbsp. of white wine vinegar
- Zest from 2 limes
- 2 tbsp. lime juice
- 1 clove of garlic, pressed
- ½ tsp of chili powder
- ¼ tsp of salt
- ½ tsp of paprika
- ¼ tsp of stevia
- 1 tbsp. of cilantro

For Chicken:
- 1 ½ tbsp. of butter
- ½ pound of chicken breast, cut into bite-sized pieces

For Aioli:
- 3 tbsp. of mayo
- Zest from lime
- 1 tsp of lime juice
- ½ a tsp of finely chopped cilantro
- 1 garlic clove, pressed

For Lettuce Wraps:
- 3 large lettuce leaves

Instructions:

In a medium-sized bowl, add all of the marinade ingredients together and blend them together until you feel they are evenly incorporated. Put the small cuts of chicken into a dish for marinating. Pour the marinated mixture over the chicken and make sure all sides of the chicken pieces have been coated evenly. Cover the dish and put in the fridge for 1–2 hours to marinate. In a saucepan, melt the butter on low heat. Once the butter is completely melted, add in the marinated chicken and turn to medium-high heat. Allow the chicken to brown on one side before flipping it to another side. The chicken can be cooked in different batches, also. For the aioli, combine all ingredients into a small bowl until evenly mixed together. Next, take your lettuce leaves and dispense chicken evenly on each leaf with a spoon. On top of the chicken, place the desired amount of aioli sauce. Serve, and enjoy!

Keto Philly Cheesesteak Omelet (4.9g carbs per two omelets)

Ingredients:
- 4 large eggs
- 2 tbsp. of olive oil
- 1 ounce of yellow onion, sliced
- ½ medium green bell pepper, sliced
- ¼ pound shaved ribeye
- 1 tsp salt
- ½ tsp of pepper
- 2 ounces of provolone cheese, sliced thin

Instructions:
Gently whisk eggs and ½ of the olive oil in a medium bowl. Heat a medium non-stick skillet and pour half of the egg mixture into it. Cover until the egg is cooked all of the ways through. Use a spatula to release the edges of the omelet from the skillet and put on a plate. Repeat the same process with the rest of the egg mix. Once the other egg is done, pour rest of the olive oil into the same skillet. Pour in sliced green peppers and onions into the pan. Cook on a medium heat until onions begin to caramelize, and the green peppers turn soft. Remove these items from the pan and set them aside. Season the ribeye with salt and pepper. Sauté meat over medium heat or until cooked all the way through. Add pepper and onion mixture back into the pan with the meat to heat back up if necessary. Take your omelet shells and layer provolone cheese and the hot mixture of meat and veggies on top. Serve, and enjoy!

Zucchini Crust Grilled Cheese

Ingredients:
- 4 cups of zucchini, shredded
- 1 large egg
- ½ cup of shredded mozzarella cheese
- 4 tbsp. of grated parmesan cheese
- 1 tsp dried oregano
- ½ tsp of salt
- Black pepper
- 1 tbsp. of butter
- 1/3 cup of shredded cheddar cheese, room temperature

Instructions:
Heat your oven to 450 degrees. Place a rack in the middle of the oven. Line a large baking sheet with parchment paper and grease it with butter, liberally. Place zucchini in microwave on high for six minutes. Once it is done, transfer it to a tea towel and squeeze out as much liquid as you can. This is super important because if you don't drain the zucchini, you'll end up with a mushy grilled cheese. It becomes almost impossible to use as slices of bread. In a large bowl, mix zucchini, egg, mozzarella cheese, parmesan cheese, oregano, salt, and pepper (to taste). Spread the zucchini mixture onto the lined baking sheet and shape it into four squares. Bake the zucchini for 15–20 minutes or until the squares become lightly brown. Remove from the oven and let it cool for about 10 minutes. Be careful during this step, you don't want to break the bread. Heat a skillet over medium heat. Butter one side of each of the zucchini bread. Place one slice of bread in the pan, buttered side down. Sprinkle with cheese. Place another slice of zucchini bread on top, buttered side up. Cook until golden brown on the first side. Flip and do the same with the other side. Each side should brown in 2–4 minutes. Cut, serve and enjoy!

Quick Dinner Recipes

Broiled Salmon (<1g carb per 1 oz. of salmon)

Ingredients:
- 4 (4 oz.) salmon filets
- 1 tbsp. of grainy mustard
- 2 cloves garlic, finely minced
- 1 tbsp. finely minced shallots
- 2 tsp finely chopped thyme leaves
- 2 tsp fresh rosemary
- Juice of half of a lemon
- Salt, to taste
- Pepper, to taste
- Lemon slices, for serving

Instructions:
Heat broiler and line a large baking pan with parchment paper. Place salmon on the pan. In a small bowl mix together the ingredients (mustard, garlic, shallots, thyme, rosemary, lemon juice, salt, and pepper). Spread mixture all over salmon fillets. Broil 7–8 minutes. Garnish with lemon slices and fresh thyme (if you'd like) and serve. Enjoy!

Taco Cheese Cups (1g carb per cup)

Ingredients:
- 3 ½ cups of shredded cheddar cheese
- 1 tbsp. of extra virgin olive oil
- 1 onion, chopped
- 3 cloves of garlic, minced
- 1 pound of ground beef
- 1 tsp chili powder
- ½ tsp ground cumin
- ½ tsp paprika
- Salt
- Chopped tomatoes, for serving
- Diced avocado, for serving
- Sour cream, for serving
- Chopped cilantro, for serving

Instructions:
First, preheat the oven the 375 degrees. Line a large baking pan with parchment paper. Put tablespoons of cheddar cheese in a small pile on the baking sheet. Bake until the cheese becomes bubbly and the edges become golden. Let them cool for a minute after removing from the over. Grease the bottom of a muffin pan and carefully peel the cheese off of the parchment paper. Place them inside the muffin tins. Let them cool for about ten minutes. In a large skillet, heat on medium, heat up the extra virgin olive oil. Add the onions and let them sauté for about five minutes, or until they become soft and slightly transparent. Add the garlic and ground beef next. Cook the beef until it is no longer pink. This will take about 6 or 7 minutes. Once that is done, drain the beef and place it back in the skillet. Add the paprika, cumin, chili powder, and salt. Transfer the cheese cups to a serving plate. Fill them with the ground beef, then add the tomatoes, sour cream, avocado, and cilantro. Serve, and enjoy!

Chicken Zucchini Alfredo (4g net carbs per serving)

Ingredients:
- 3 large zucchinis
- 2 tbsp. extra virgin olive oil
- ¾ pounds of chicken breast
- Salt
- Pepper
- 1 tsp Italian seasoning
- 2 cloves of garlic, finely minced
- ¾ cup half and half
- 4oz cream cheese
- ½ cup of freshly grated parmesan
- ¼ cup of chopped parsley

Instructions:
Make zucchini "pappardelle." Using a vegetable peeler, peel the zucchinis to make long, thin strips. Lay them on a paper-towel-lined baking sheet until ready to use them. On medium heat, place the chicken breast and one tablespoon of extra virgin olive oil in a large skillet and let it cook 6–8 minutes on each side. Season each side of the chicken with salt, pepper, and Italian seasoning. Transfer the chicken to a cutting board. Slice it into strips. Add the remaining tablespoon of extra virgin olive oil to the skillet. Add the garlic and cook it until it becomes fragrant. This usually takes about a minute. From there, add the half and a half and the cream cheese to the skillet. Stir this often until the cream cheese becomes melted. Add in the freshly grated parmesan, season with salt and pepper. Wait for the sauce to thicken (about 3 to 5 minutes). Finally, fold in the chicken and zucchini pappardelle. Add the parsley last. Serve and enjoy immediately!

Easy Turkey Chili (5.5g carbs)

Ingredients:
- 1 tbsp. of virgin olive oil
- 1 yellow onion, diced
- 1 small green pepper, diced
- 2 cloves of minced garlic
- 2 pounds of ground turkey breast
- 1.5 tbsp. of chili powder
- 1 tsp of garlic powder
- 1 tbsp. ground cumin
- 1 tsp cayenne powder
- 1 cup low carb tomato sauce
- Salt and pepper, to taste
- Shredded cheddar cheese, for serving
- Sour cream, for serving

Instructions:

Heat a large skillet with the olive oil in it. Heat should be on medium high. Add in the diced onions and peppers and sauté until they are browned. This should take about 3–4 minutes. Stir in the garlic and cook for about another minute or so. Add in the ground turkey and season it with salt and pepper. Cook the turkey until it is completely browned and then add in the other seasonings. Stir in the tomato sauce and season to taste if what you have already added is not enough. Simmer on low heat for ten minutes. Serve with shredded cheese and sour cream. Enjoy!

Advice

Beginning the Keto diet can be really hard, especially if it is already hard for you to find time to eat a good, nutritional meal. But before you inlay the idea, look up some success stories. See how other women in your position have successfully done Keto and managed to keep everything else intact. It makes your journey a lot easier. You can also ask for help. Having someone support your journey—maybe a spouse or your children—can push you to do your absolute best. It helps keep you motivated!

A lot of women revolve their Keto diets around foods that they know they love. I think the love of pizza, cheeseburgers, and pasta are a common factor between us all. The good thing about these and many other foods is that there is a Keto-version of them. You can have foods you really want and still eat healthily. If we could all make the switch, I think we would be surprised at how good the food really is.

Another great way to be at your *Keto-best* is to connect with people on social media. Putting yourself out there is a little intimidating, but you would be surprised at how many people are going through the same thing you are going through. You both could help each other out. Talking about what problems you are having warrants an array of answers from people all over the world. Within those people, there could be someone who is just like you–boost each other up and get healthy!

Women Who Gladly Shared Their Keto Stories Online

Allison, 41, lost 25lbs in 6 months: Find some high-protein recipes you love!
"My current favorite is stuffed peppers with ground beef and melted mozzarella. And low carb desserts are key! They kept me from feeling deprived. I used resources like Keto cookbooks."

Esther, lost 41lbs in 5 months: Eat at least 50 grams of protein a day!

"In the past, diets have left me crazy-hungry. Now, I maintain a caloric deficit, but I do it while making sure I have enough fat, protein, and fiber, which keeps me satisfied."

Joanna, 33, lost 60lbs in a year: Eat the Keto-friendly foods that you legit enjoy!
"I built my diet around foods that I really like: Caesar salads, cheese, and chicken wings. I stopped feeling guilty about eating them (which I did in the past because they're high in fat) and now I actually take pleasure in the food that I'm eating. The best part is that my cravings have pretty much stopped."

Success stories are everywhere! You have the potential to be one of them—if you want to. The most important thing to remember is that your body is the most important thing. If your body isn't happy, you aren't either. Listen to what your body is telling you. Also, don't fear away because of myths! Our bodies used to run perfectly fine, as they would on the Keto diet—way, way, way back in the day. The Keto diet is designed around how the first people lived without a grocery store or farming. All they had to eat was what they could find. Hence, if they didn't hunt and gather, they didn't eat. If they got a rabbit, they would fuel their bodies with what fat, protein, and fiber they could gain that. Sometimes, they would have to go days without eating, and that is why intermittent fasting is an intricate detail of the Keto diet. You will function normally on this diet, but be aware of the Keto flu. It is short-lived, but it can take its toll on your body. There are steps to help you get past it easier.

- Some advice to get through the Keto flu is to eat an excessive amount of fat for the first week or so. Let your body know things are changing!
- Don't restrict calories! Eat until you are not hungry anymore.
- Keto or Fasting-Choose one to start! You don't have to do both, and you definitely don't have to stick with whichever is not working for you.
- If you make fat bombs, make them as nutrient-dense as possible.

- Don't be hard on yourself if you don't meet your daily goals.
- Be aware of the low-protein slippery slope—high levels of Ketones don't mean much if you are losing muscle instead of fat.
- Create a rewards system—if you make your macros for a couple of days, maybe have an extra fat bomb the next morning!
- Don't treat yourself with a cheat day! This is a big one. Having one cheat day will not be worth the body being knocked out of Ketosis. It will be like going through the Keto flu all over again once you get back on track. Reward with fats, not carbs!
- Set realistic goals, not ones that will make you feel like you need to be punished for not reaching them.
- Track everything you put into your body!
- Add in exercise if you feel like doing so!

There are a number of different ways to keep yourself on track. Do your best if the Keto diet is for you. If it isn't right now, that is okay. Maybe come back to it at another time. If you are wanting a weight change or wanting an immediate change to how you feel, the Keto diet could be a perfect fit. If you find yourself getting bored, switch up your meal plans! Maybe creating new goals for yourself. Experience the lifestyle change that is the Ketogenic diet. You'll be glad you did!

Here is a beginner's food list. These are the essential products you'll need to begin Keto. They are high in fat, protein, and low in carbs. Some of them are used purely for the cooking method.

- Salmon
- Sardines
- Cod liver oil
- Eggs
- Grass-fed beef
- Grass-fed butter
- Grass-fed ghee

- Hemp seeds
- Chia Seeds
- Flax seeds
- Stevia
- Allulose
- Monk fruit
- Erythritol
- Spinach
- Zucchini
- Broccoli
- Cauliflower
- Lettuce
- Mushrooms
- Kale
- Garlic
- Celery
- Blackberries
- Raspberries
- Strawberries
- Avocados
- Eggplant
- Squash
- Lemon
- Lime
- Tomatoes
- Olives
- Peppers
- Cucumbers
- Coconut
- Cheese
- Heavy whipping cream
- Cream cheese
- Sour cream
- Plain Greek yogurt
- Nut milk
- Cottage cheese

- Olive oil
- Avocado oil
- MCT oil
- MCT powder
- Coconut oil
- Walnut oil
- Ricotta
- Wild-caught seafood
- Wild-caught game
- Uncured bacon
- Bone Broth
- Apple cider vinegar
- Dark chocolate (high percentage of cocoa)

This is, by all means, not a complete list of grocery items for Keto. But most of these items will get you started. Make sure you read labels before you purchase these items. Some products have additives to make the products last longer. You want the most whole foods you can get. Also, watch out for sugar alcohols!

This may look like an expensive list—and depending on where you live, it might be. However, the good news about this list is that it can last you for a long time. For example, buying a box of stevia or buying any of the cooking oils is going to last you for more than one meal. It can actually last weeks! Other things—you can divide up. Ground-fed beef can be stretched out for a couple of meals. If you and your family are fans of leftovers, you can really stretch it out. Things like heavy whipping cream—you might have to purchase more often, as it gets consumed pretty quickly. Other things like the leafy greens and berries are more of the same. But luckily, you are on Keto, and you will be consuming them rather quickly to meet your macros! A typical day of eating a standard Keto diet can look like this:

Breakfast:
- 3 large eggs cooked with grass-fed butter
- 1 medium avocado topped with sea salt
- 4oz of smoked salmon
- Ghee – 2 tbsp.

Lunch:
- 1 can of tuna
- Raw spinach with two tablespoons of olive oil
- Raw almonds

Dinner:
- 1 tablespoon of butter
- 2 cups of mushrooms
- Grilled chicken leg with skin

These items will use a lot of the products you bought on your list. You will also have a lot of leftovers to use for your next meal. Hence, while the first shopping trip might be a bit expensive, it won't stay that way. The next few trips to the store will be to replenish your vegetables and dairy-based products. This typical day will also differ a bit depending on your macros. Therefore, this may work for some people—but if your goals on Keto are different, you may need to increase fat intake a bit more or maybe consume a bit more protein. It also depends on which Keto diet you are doing. If you are, for example, doing the high-protein Ketogenic diet, then your protein intake will be a lot higher than a person who is doing a standard Ketogenic diet (SKD). If you are on a CKD, then your carb intake will be higher. The same goes for a TKD, which allows for more carbs based on your workouts.

Conclusion

Thank you for making it through to the end of Keto Diet for Women: Beginner's Guide to Loss Weight Fast. Let's hope it was informative and able to provide you with all of the tools you need to achieve your goals—whatever they may be.

The next step is to determine if the Ketogenic Lifestyle is for you. If it is, please refer to this audiobook as your one-stop information shop. Everything that you need to know is here! If you are a woman who is premenopausal, suffering from type II diabetes, or just want to lose weight—your answers are here. There are essential details on how to go through the Keto diet as a woman. You'll find great, easy recipes to start your new life with as well as some key snacks that will help you make it through the day. It's all here!

Thank you.

CPSIA information can be obtained
at www.ICGtesting.com
Printed in the USA
BVHW041115100720
583432BV00010B/104

9 781648 661785